Mosby's
Anatomy
Coloring Book

Mosby's

Anatomy Coloring Book

Edited by

Barbara A. Magerl, RN, BSN, MS
President,
Specialized Medical Education and Training, Inc.
Munster, Indiana

Bernadette A. Sanner, RN, BSN, MS
Director, Clinical Services
Care Center Inc.
Evanston, Illinois

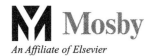

An Affiliate of Elsevier

11830 Westline Industrial Drive
St. Louis, Missouri 63146

NOTICE

Nursing is an ever-changing field. Standard safety precautions must be followed, but as new research and clinical experience broaden our knowledge, changes in treatment and drug therapy may become necessary or appropriate. Readers are advised to check the most current product information provided by the manufacturer of each drug to be administered to verify the recommended dose, the method and duration of administration, and contraindications. It is the responsibility of the licensed prescriber, relying on experience and knowledge of the patient, to determine dosages and the best treatment for each individual patient. Neither the publisher nor the author assumes any liability for any injury and/or damage to persons or property arising from this publication.

ISBN-13: 978-0-323-01971-2
ISBN-10: 0-323-01971-4

Executive Vice President, Nursing and Health Professions: Sally Schrefer
Senior Editor: Tom Wilhelm
Senior Developmental Editor: Jeff Downing
Publishing Services Manager: Catherine Albright Jackson
Project Manager: Celeste Clingan
Design Coordinator: Amy Buxton

Printed in USA

Last digit is the print number: 9 8 7 6 5 4

CONTENTS

INTRODUCTION

Anatomy is the study of bones, muscles, blood vessels, and organs of the body. It can be overwhelming if not studied from simple to more complex. If you learn the basic structures well, you will see how the parts of the body fit and work together. This book has been developed to enable the student to begin the journey of studying anatomy in a simple, positive manner.

Use this book in its prescribed format and you will find an easy way to enhance your knowledge. This book will help you to visually understand the parts of each system and how they build on each other. We expect you to use your anatomy textbook for reference so that you not only identify the structures properly, spell them correctly but also color the organs as they are identified.

We will allow you to choose the colors you wish, but odds are that if a doctor would see the colors you choose he or she would be greatly surprised. This is because the color of the organs in the human body provide important clues about the presence of disease. For example, a yellow liver is full of fat, a red liver is full of blood, a green liver is full of bile.

In reality, our internal organs are not very colorful but in this instance, color them the way you wish, have fun, and explore.

ACKNOWLEDGEMENTS

The editors of this book are indebted to many people who helped make this book happen. The sales staff who called on us and discussed the need for a book that covered the simple areas and got us started in this first endeavor. The Developmental Editors who so patiently worked with us, listened to our ideas, and guided us through the entire process. A special nod goes to the illustrators who worked so diligently on our rough sketches (and we do mean rough sketches).

UNIT 1 The Skin

FIGURE **1-1** LAYERS OF THE SKIN

The figure below illustrates the skin (integumentary) system, the largest organ of the body, on a structural basis comprised of three parts. The figure below depicts a longitudinal section of the skin. The skin layers are bracketed on the right of the figure. Identify these layers by name and color each of the structures below in a different color.

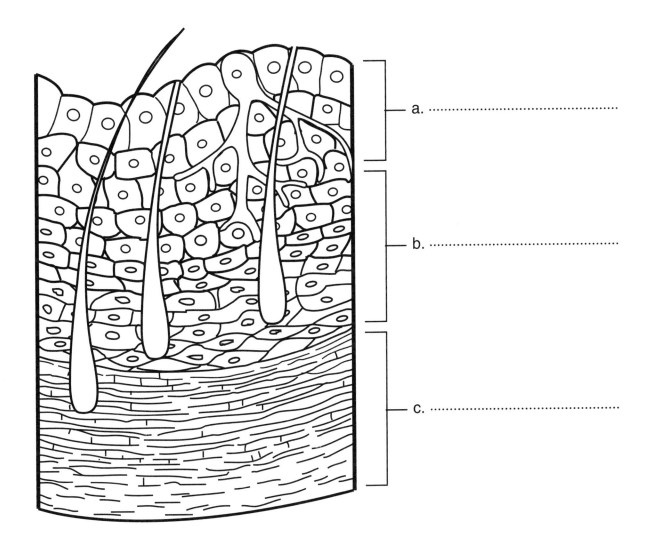

a. ....

b. ....

c. ....

UNIT 1 The Skin

FIGURE **1–2 ACCESSORY ORGANS OF THE SKIN**
The figure below depicts a longitudinal section of the skin. Many accessory organs are found within the skin. In the picture below identify and color the structures indicated with a line.

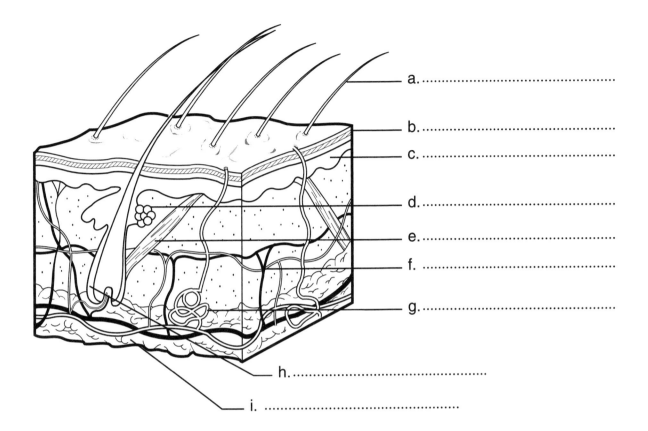

a. ....

b. ....

c. ....

d. ....

e. ....

f. ....

g. ....

h. ....

i. ....

FIGURE 2–1 TYPES OF BONES

The figure below depicts a frontal view of the skeleton. Five types of bones are indicated by lines. On each line, identify the bone type. Color the bone a different color once identified.

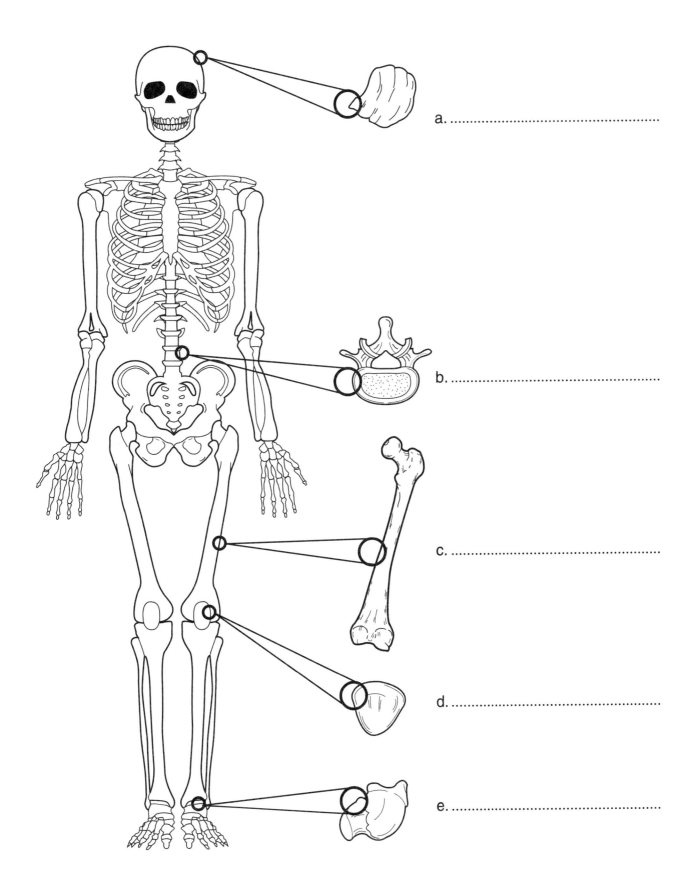

a. ....

b. ....

c. ....

d. ....

e. ....

8

FIGURE 2-2 BONE STRUCTURE

The figure below illustrates the makeup of bones. Identify the structures that are labeled with a blank line and color each structure with a different color.

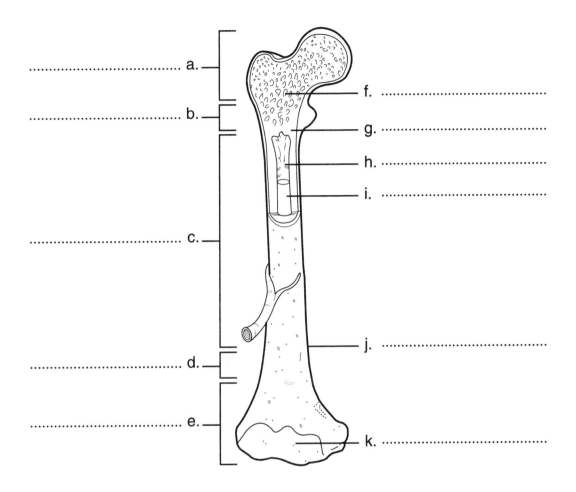

a. ....

b. ....

c. ....

d. ....

e. ....

f. ....

g. ....

h. ....

i. ....

j. ....

k. ....

UNIT 2 The Skeletal System

FIGURE **2–3** **SKULL (Lateral View)**
The figure below depicts a lateral view of the skull. Identify the various areas of the skull and color each with a different color. Correct spelling of the words is as important as the color identification.

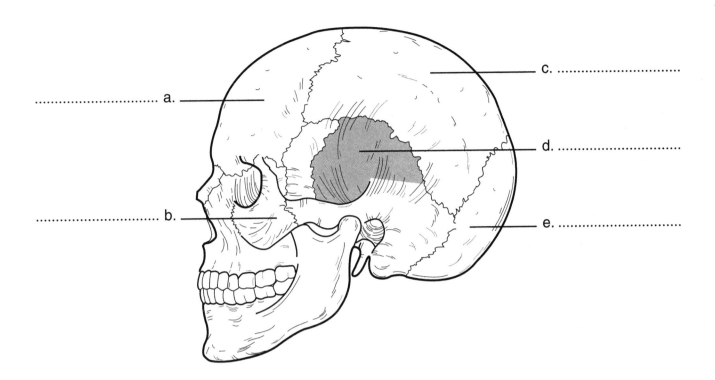

UNIT 2 The Skeletal System

FIGURE **2–4** **SKULL (Cranium)**
The figure below depicts a cranial view of the skull. Many structures are located within the skull. Identify and color those structures selected by the lines. Spelling is important.

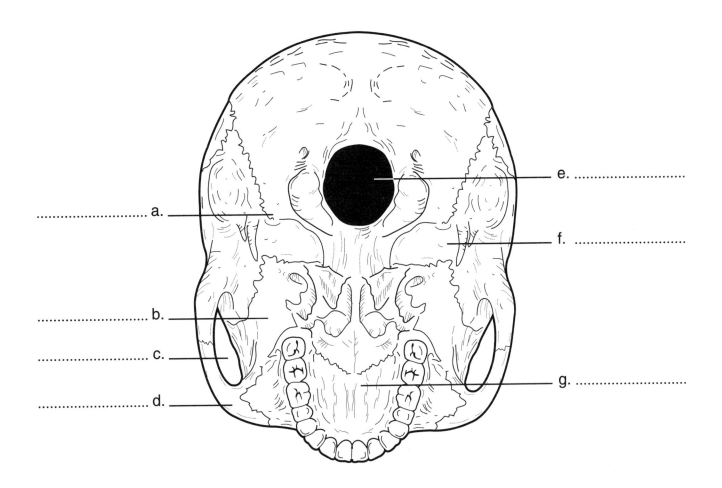

a. ....

b. ....

c. ....

d. ....

e. ....

f. ....

g. ....

FIGURE 2–5 FACIAL BONES
The figure below depicts the facial bones. Identify and color those structures selected by lines.

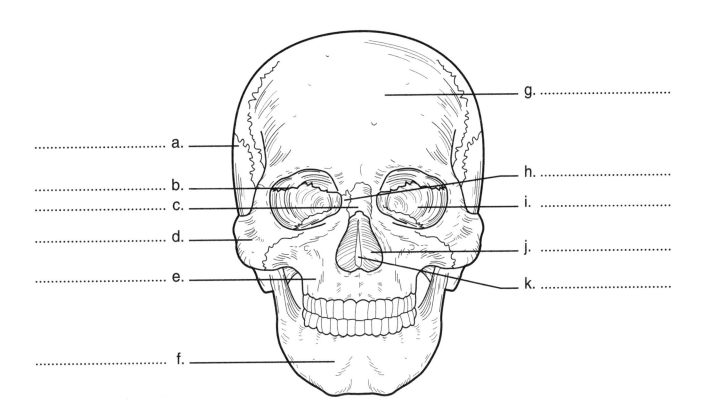

.... a.

.... b.

.... c.

.... d.

.... e.

.... f.

g. ....

h. ....

i. ....

j. ....

k. ....

UNIT 2 The Skeletal System

FIGURE **2–6** **VERTEBRAL SECTIONS (Cervical, Thoracic, Lumbar, and Sacral)**
The figure below depicts a lateral view of the spine. The sections of the spine are indicated by brackets. Identify the sections by name and color each structure identified with a different color. Numbers 1, 2, and 3 are specifically named vertebral bodies. Identify them individually.

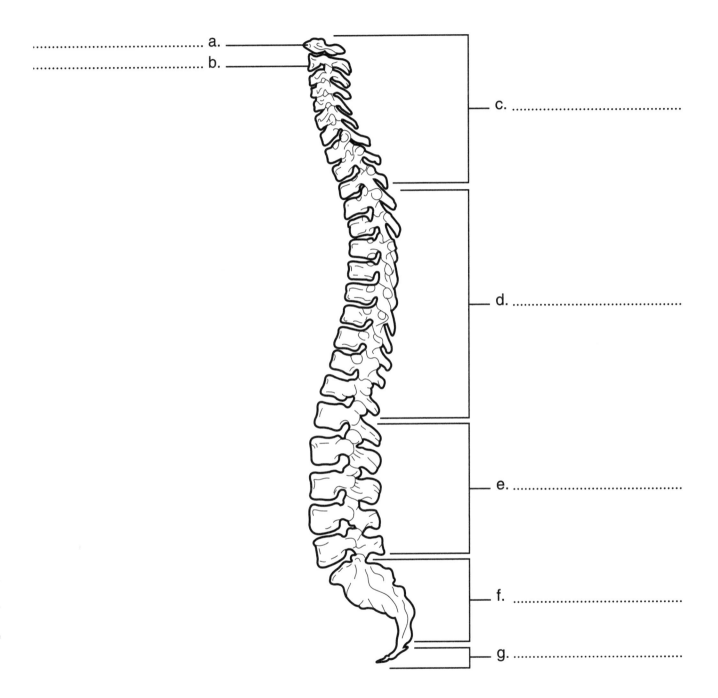

.... a. ____

.... b. ____

c. ....

d. ....

e. ....

f. ....

g. ....

FIGURE **2–7** **VERTEBRAL SECTIONS (Various Types)**
The figure below depicts superior views of the four types of vertebrae. Identify each type by name and color each one with a different color.

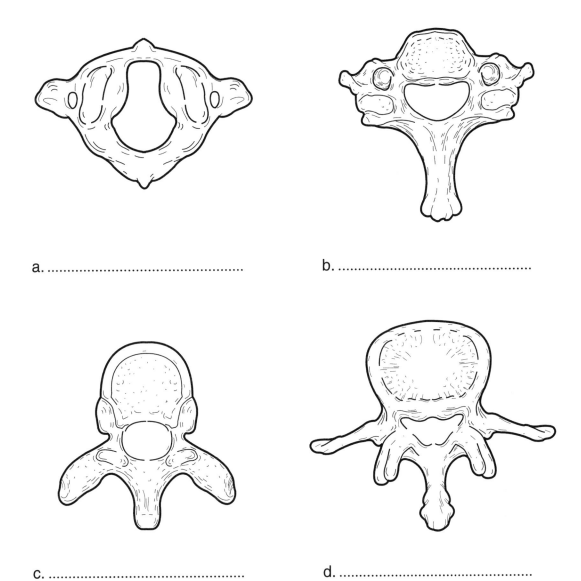

a. ....

b. ....

c. ....

d. ....

FIGURE 2–8 THORAX (Sternum, Ribs & False Ribs, and Cartilage)
The figure below depicts the various areas of the thorax. Identify each section marked by its name, and color each section with a different color.

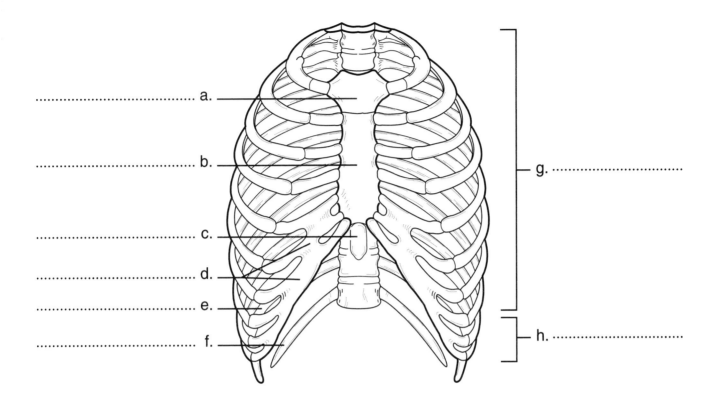

.... a. _____

.... b. _____

.... c. _____

.... d. _____

.... e. _____

.... f. _____

g. ....

h. ....

FIGURE 2–9 PECTORAL GIRDLE (Clavicle and Scapula) AND UPPER LIMB
Below is a diagram of an entire upper limb. Identify each structure indicated by the lines, and select a different color for each structure.

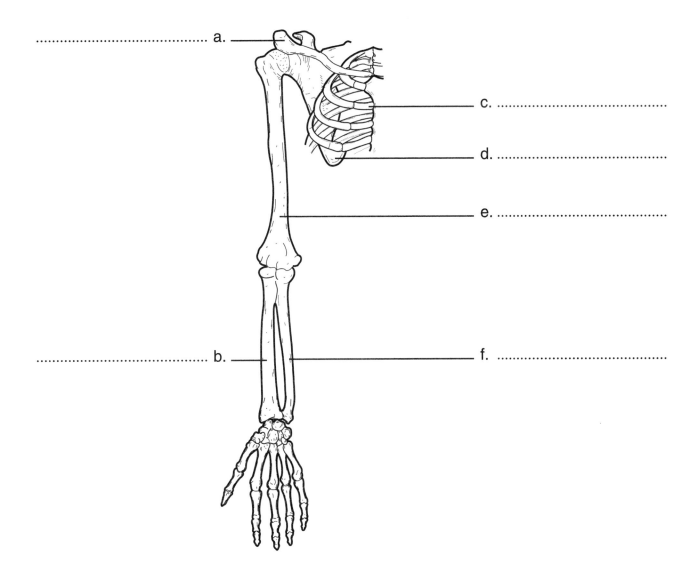

a. ....

c. ....

d. ....

e. ....

b. ....

f. ....

UNIT 2 The Skeletal System

FIGURES **2–10** (Anterior View) and **2–11** (Posterior View) BONES OF THE HAND
The diagram below is a detailed picture of the hands. Identify the structures indicated by the lines and brackets, and color each a different color.

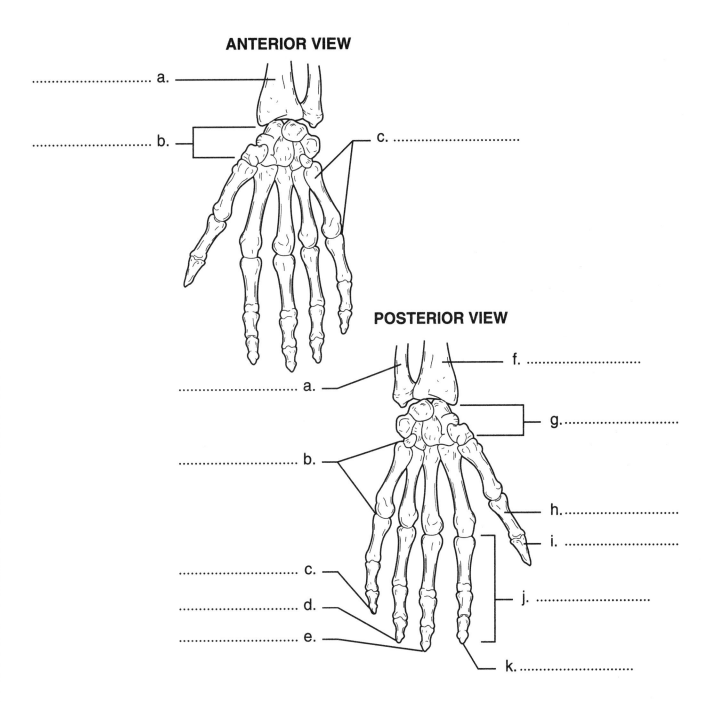

ANTERIOR VIEW

.... a.

.... b.

c. ....

POSTERIOR VIEW

.... a.

f. ....

g. ....

.... b.

h. ....

i. ....

.... c.

.... d.

j. ....

.... e.

k. ....

FIGURE **2–12** PELVIC GIRDLE
The figure below depicts anterior and posterior views of the pelvic girdle. Identify each section marked by its name, and color each section with a different color.

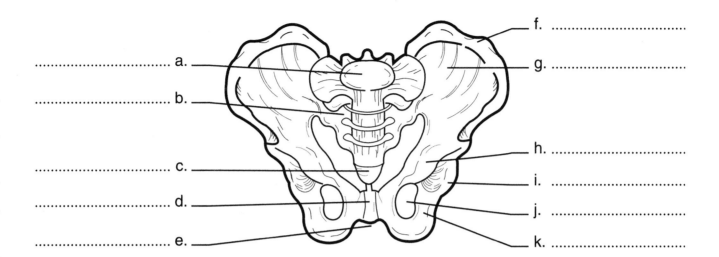

a. ....

b. ....

c. ....

d. ....

e. ....

f. ....

g. ....

h. ....

i. ....

j. ....

k. ....

FIGURES 2–13 LOWER LIMBS (Anterior and Posterior Views)
The figure below depicts both the anterior and posterior views of the bones of the lower leg. Identify each structure, and select different colors for each structure identified.

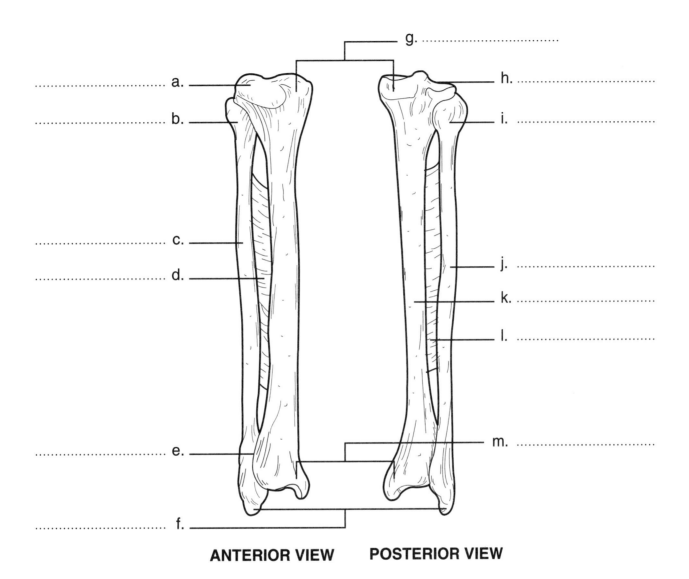

g. ....

a. ....   h. ....

b. ....   i. ....

c. ....   j. ....

d. ....   k. ....

l. ....

e. ....   m. ....

f. ....

ANTERIOR VIEW   POSTERIOR VIEW

FIGURES **2–14** (Anterior View) and **2–15** (Posterior View) LOWER LIMBS (Bones of the legs)
The diagram below depicts a lateral view of the bones of the leg. Select different colors for each structure you identify.

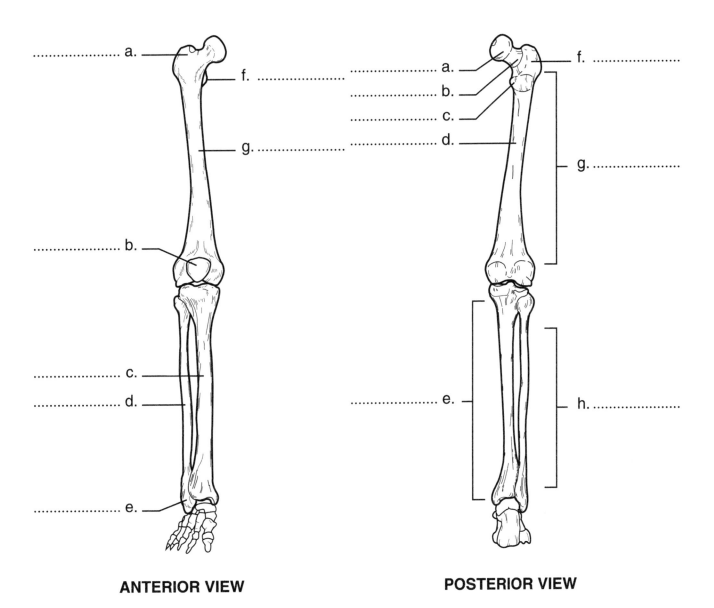

ANTERIOR VIEW

POSTERIOR VIEW

FIGURE 2–16 BONES OF THE FOOT

The figure below depicts a lateral view of the bones of the foot. Select a different color for each structure as you identify it.

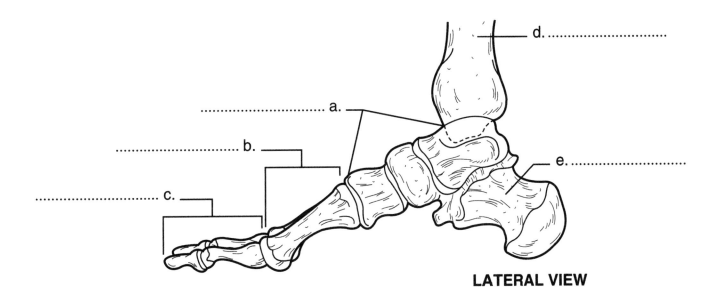

d. ....

a. ....

b. ....

c. ....

e. ....

LATERAL VIEW

FIGURE **2–17** **STRUCTURES OF THE KNEE**

The figure below depicts an anterior view of the structures of the knee. Select a different color for each structure as you identify it.

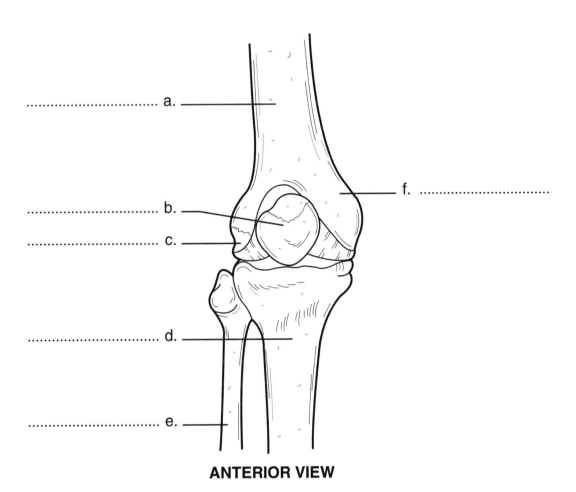

a. ....

b. ....

c. ....

d. ....

e. ....

f. ....

ANTERIOR VIEW

UNIT 2 The Skeletal System

FIGURE 2-18 JOINTS

The pictures below depict various types of joints in the body. Each type is presently identified as an immovable joint, a slightly movable joint, or a freely movable joint. These are not their proper names. Identify each joint by its proper name, and color joint identified.

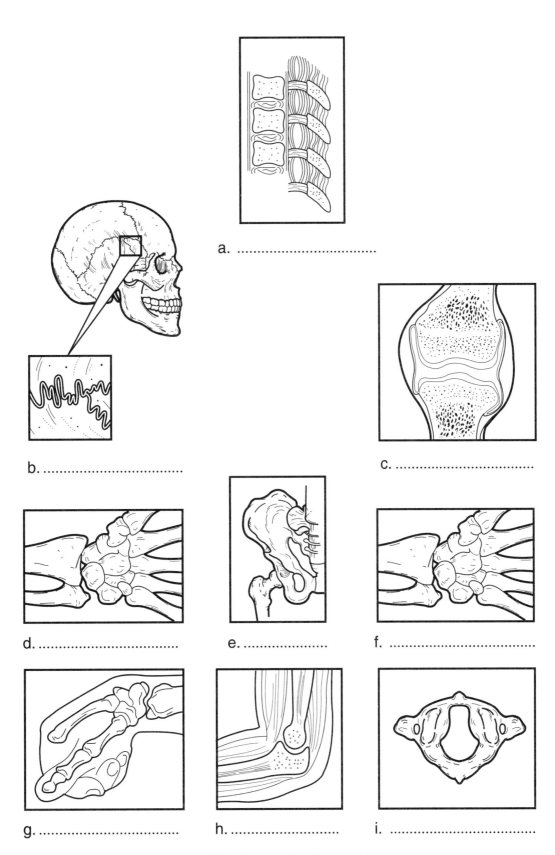

a. ....

b. ....

c. ....

d. ....

e. ....

f. ....

g. ....

h. ....

i. ....

UNIT 3 The Muscular System

FIGURE 3–1 TYPES OF MUSCLES

The figure below illustrates the three basic types of muscles within the muscular system. Identify the particular type of muscle labeled with a blank line and color each structure within the muscle with a different color.

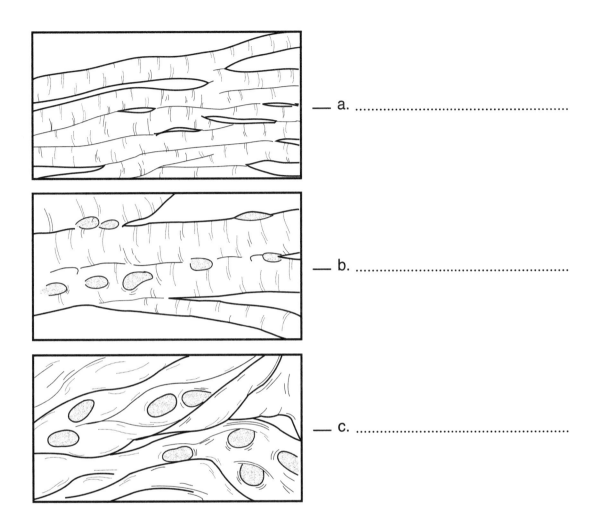

— a. ....

— b. ....

— c. ....

FIGURE 3–2 SKELETAL MUSCLES OF THE HEAD

The figure below illustrates the muscles within the head. Identify the structures that are labeled with a blank line and color each structure with a different color.

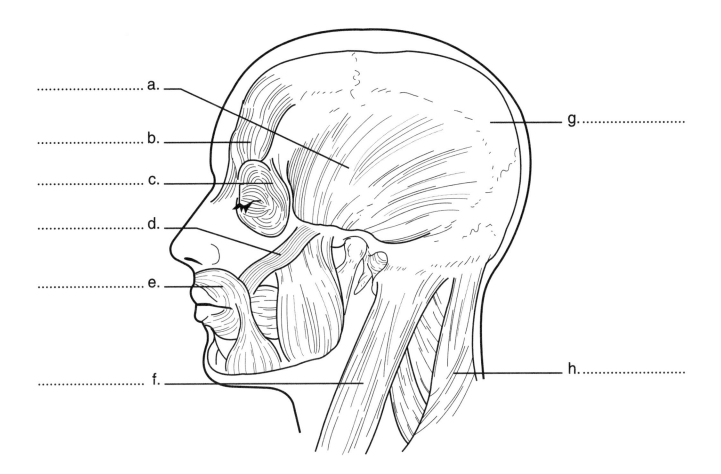

.... a.

.... b.

.... c.

.... d.

.... e.

.... f.

g. ....

h. ....

FIGURE 3–3 MUSCLES OF THE TRUNK (Anterior View)

The figure below illustrates the muscles of the trunk from the anterior view. Identify the muscles that have been marked with a blank line. Then select a color for each identified muscle and color that particular muscle.

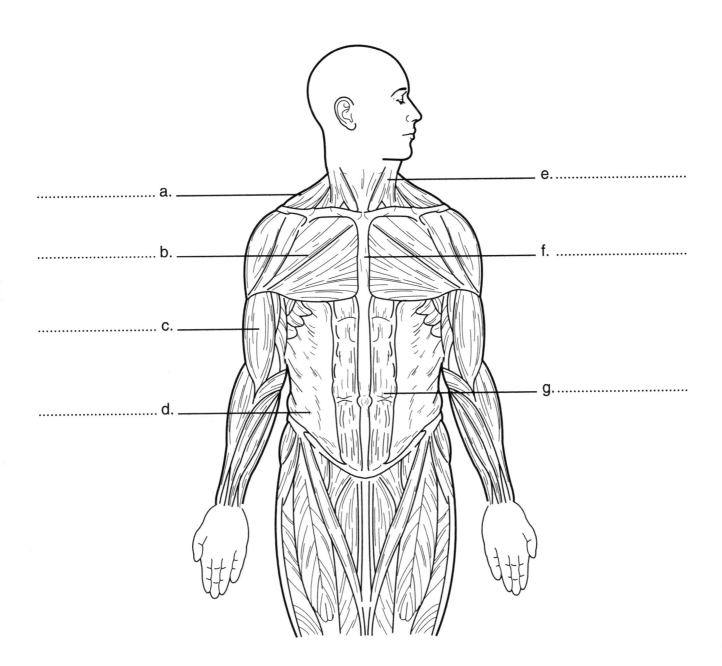

FIGURE **3–4** **MUSCLES OF THE TRUNK (Posterior View)**

The figure below illustrates the muscles of the trunk from the posterior view. Identify the muscles that have been marked with a blank line. Then select a color for each identified muscle and color that particular muscle.

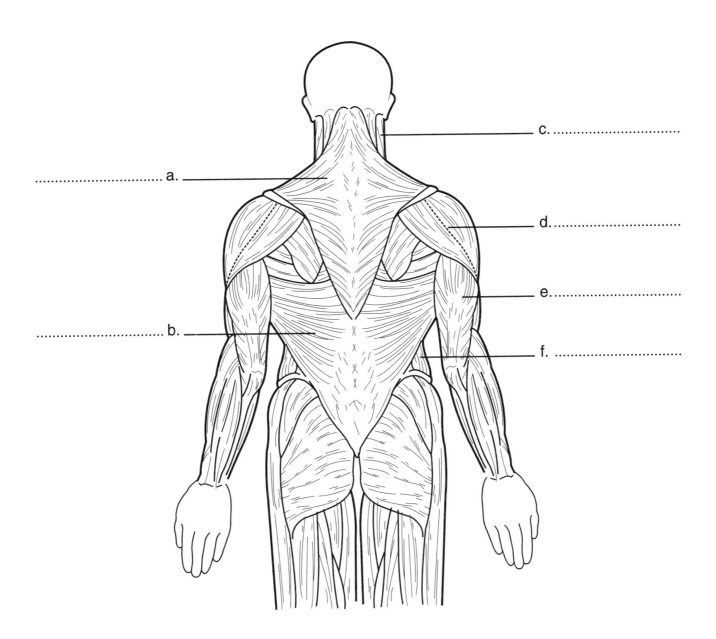

.... a.

.... b.

c. ....

d. ....

e. ....

f. ....

FIGURE 3–5 MUSCLES OF THE ARM AND FOREARM

The figure below illustrates the muscles of the arm and forearm. Identify the particular types of muscles labeled with a blank line and color each structure with a different color. Check your spelling for accuracy.

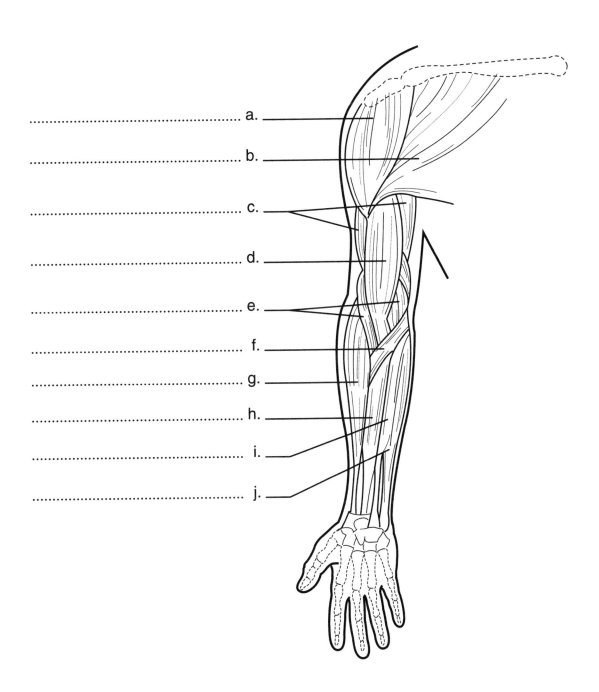

.... a.

.... b.

.... c.

.... d.

.... e.

.... f.

.... g.

.... h.

.... i.

.... j.

FIGURE **3–6** **MUSCLES OF THE HIP, THIGH, AND LEG**
The figure below illustrates the strongest muscles of the body, those of the hip, thigh, and leg. Identify the particular types of muscles labeled with a blank line and color each structure with a different color. Check your spelling for accuracy.

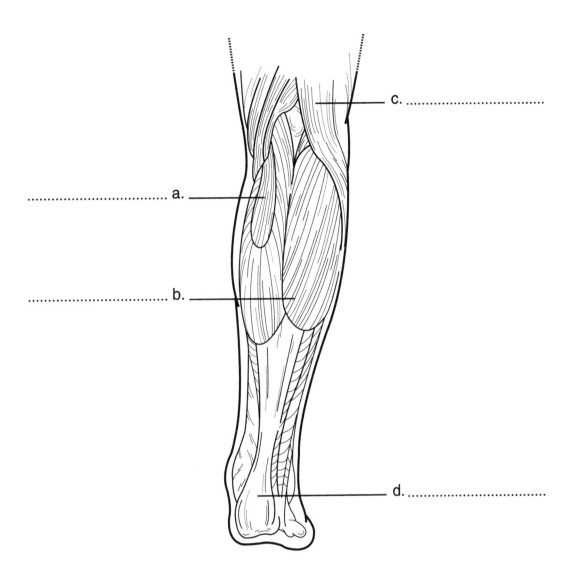

c. ....

a. ....

b. ....

d. ....

FIGURE **4–1** BASIC NEURON

The figure below illustrates the basic neuron of the nervous system. Identify the structures that are indicated with blank lines, and color each structure with a different color.

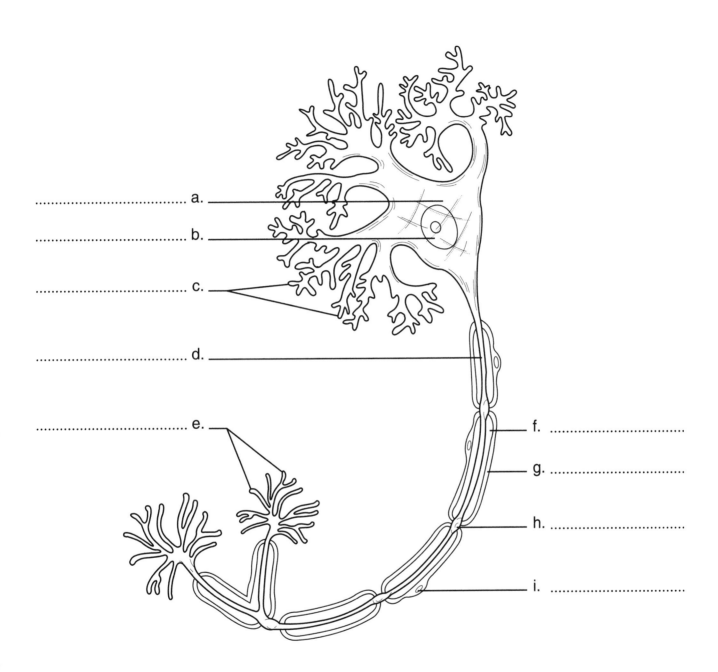

.... a. _____

.... b. _____

.... c. _____

.... d. _____

.... e. _____

f. ....

g. ....

h. ....

i. ....

FIGURE **4–2** **BRAIN (External Anatomy)**
The figure below illustrates the external anatomy of the brain, a part of the central nervous system. Identify the structures that are indicated with blank lines, and color each structure with a different color.

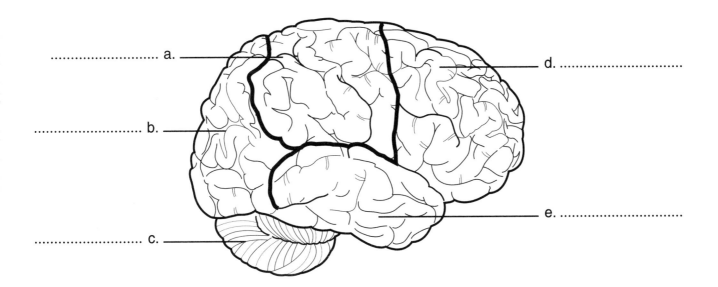

.... a. ——

.... b. ——

.... c. ——

d. ....

e. ....

UNIT 4 The Nervous System

FIGURE **4–3** BRAIN (Sagittal and Coronal Sections)
The figure below illustrates the sagittal and coronal sections of the brain within the central nervous system. Identify the structures that are indicated with blank lines, and color each structure with a different color.

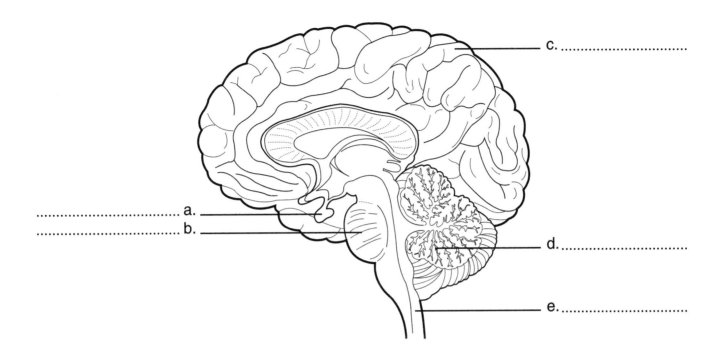

.... a. _____

.... b. _____

c. ....

d. ....

e. ....

UNIT 4 The Nervous System

FIGURE **4–4 BRAIN** (Meninges and Spinal Fluid)
The figure below illustrates the sections of the brain known as the meninges and the spinal fluid, parts of the central nervous system. Identify the structures indictated, and color each structure a different color.

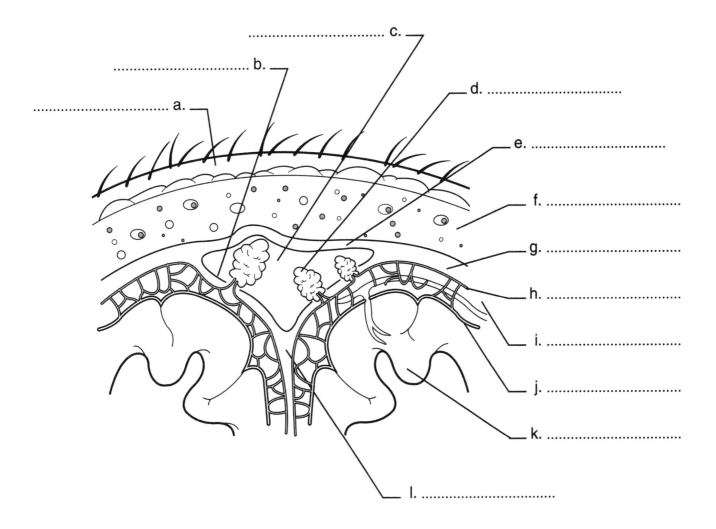

FIGURE 4–5 SPINAL CORD (Cross-Section)

The figure below illustrates cross-sections of the spinal cord, also a part of the central nervous system. Identify the structures that are indicated with blank lines, and color each structure with a different color.

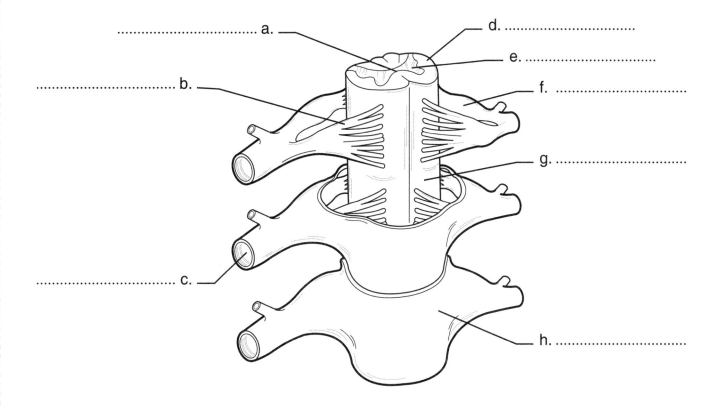

.... a.

.... b.

.... c.

d. ....

e. ....

f. ....

g. ....

h. ....

UNIT 4 The Nervous System

FIGURE **4–6** NERVES OF THE SPINE

The figure below illustrates a cross-section of the nerves of the spine. Identify the structures that are indicated with blank lines, and color each structure with a different color.

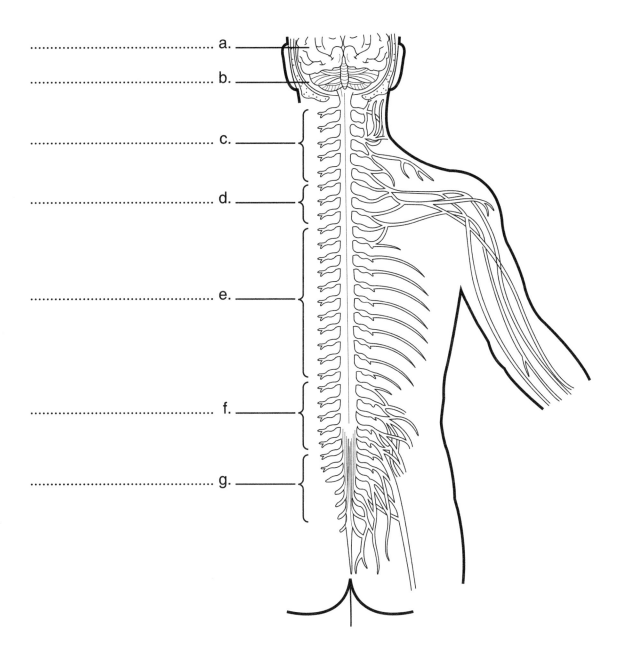

.... a. ____

.... b. ____

.... c. ____

.... d. ____

.... e. ____

.... f. ____

.... g. ____

62

UNIT 4 The Nervous System

FIGURE **4–7** CRANIAL NERVES

The figure below illustrates the cranial nerves. Cranial nerves are mixed nerves because they contain both sensory and motor fibers. Identify the individual structures that are indicated with blank lines, and color each structure with a different color.

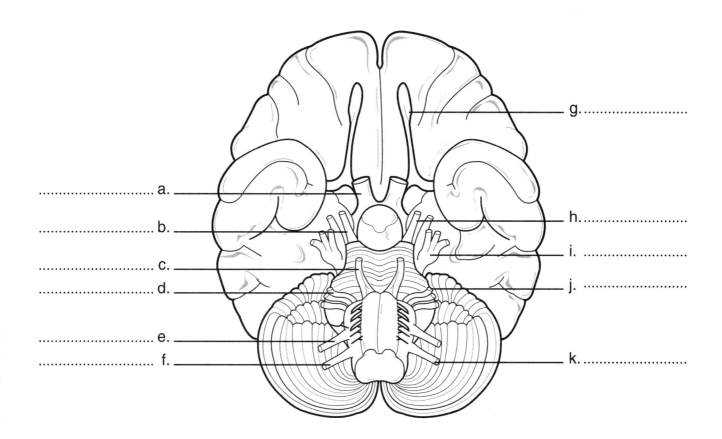

FIGURE 5–1 STRUCTURES OF THE EYE (Cross-Section)

The figure below is a sagittal section through the eye with an emphasis on the main structures. Select different colors for the structures identified by blank lines. Color the structures and fill in the blanks with the correct name.

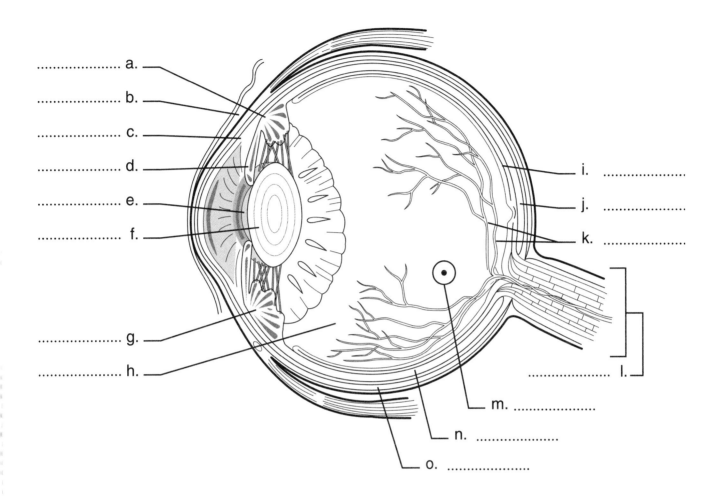

.... a.

.... b.

.... c.

.... d.

.... e.

.... f.

.... g.

.... h.

i. ....

j. ....

k. ....

l. ....

m. ....

n. ....

o. ....

FIGURES 6–1 (Inner Bones) and 6-2 (Outer Structures) STRUCTURES OF THE EAR

The figures below illustrates the inner bones of the ear. Examine closely the structures that are labeled with a blank line and identify each structure. Then color each structure you identified a different color.

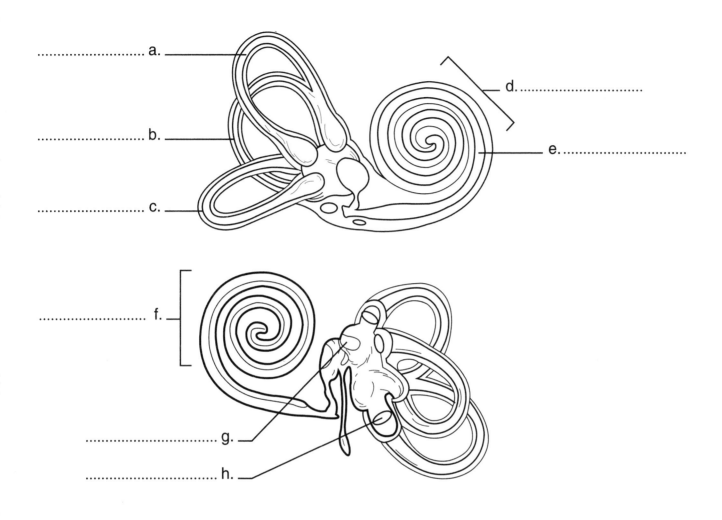

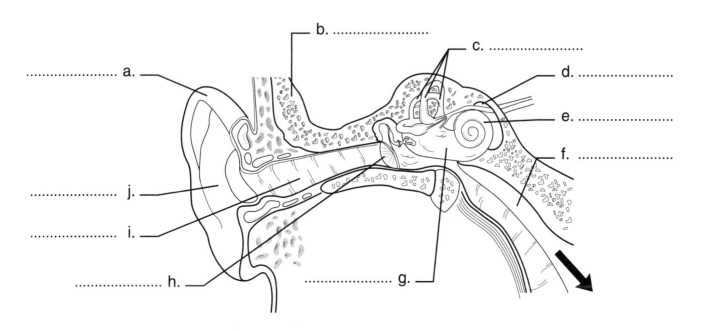

UNIT 7 Nose, Mouth, Throat

FIGURE **7-1** THE NOSE, MOUTH and THROAT

The figure below illustrates a cross section of the nose, mouth and throat. Identify the structures that are labeled with a blank line and color each structure with a different color.

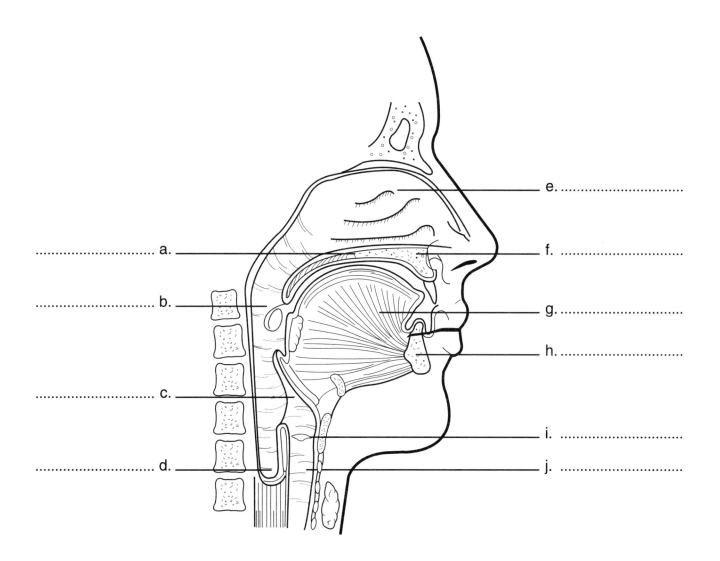

e. ....

a. ....

f. ....

b. ....

g. ....

h. ....

c. ....

i. ....

d. ....

j. ....

FIGURE **7–2** **STRUCTURES OF THE TONGUE**

The figure below illustrates a cross-section of the tongue. Identify the structures that are labeled with a blank line, keeping in mind that some areas indicate taste buds. Color in only areas of the tongue that are specific for taste.

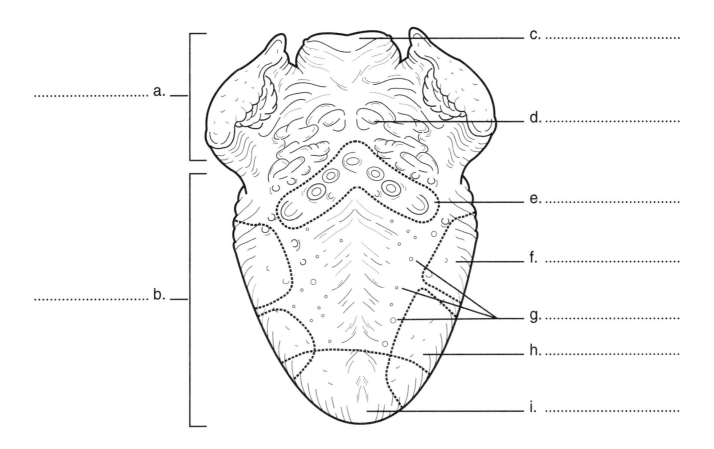

a. ....

b. ....

c. ....

d. ....

e. ....

f. ....

g. ....

h. ....

i. ....

UNIT 7 Nose, Mouth, Throat

FIGURE 7-3 THROAT STRUCTURE (Cross-section)
Pictured below is a cross-section of the throat. Identify each structure listed below by filling in the blank lines. Spelling is important. Select a different color for each corresponding figure that is identified.

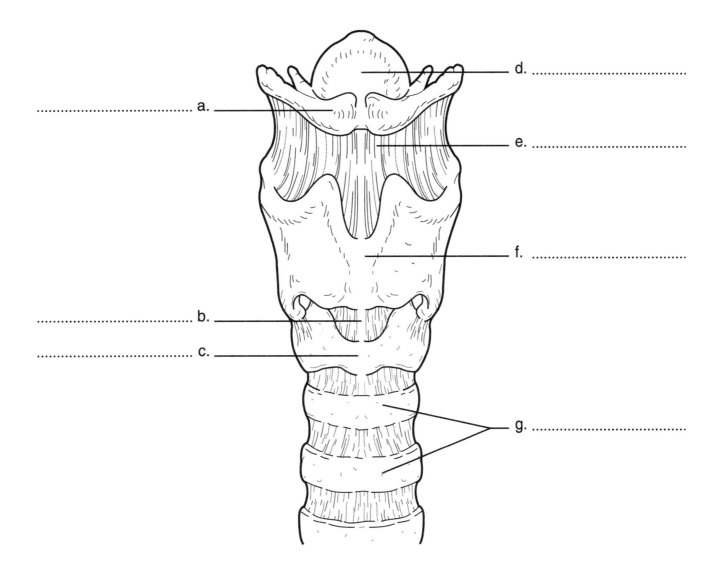

.... a. _____

.... b. _____

.... c. _____

d. ....

e. ....

f. ....

g. ....

UNIT 8 The Teeth

FIGURE **8–1** TYPES OF TEETH

The figure below illustrates a cross-section of the types of teeth. Identify the structures by groups, which are labeled with a blank line. Color each group a different color.

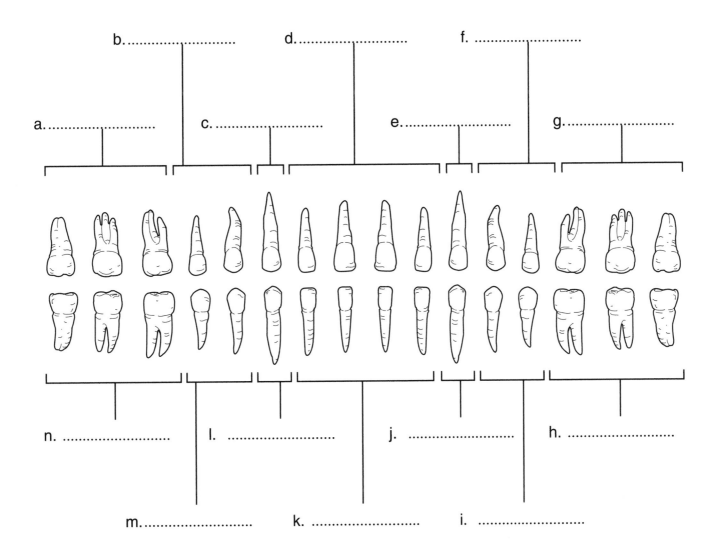

a. ....

b. ....

c. ....

d. ....

e. ....

f. ....

g. ....

h. ....

i. ....

j. ....

k. ....

l. ....

m. ....

n. ....

FIGURE **8–2** TOOTH STRUCTURE

The figure below illustrates a cross-section of a tooth. Identify the structures that are labeled with a blank line and color each identified structure with a different color.

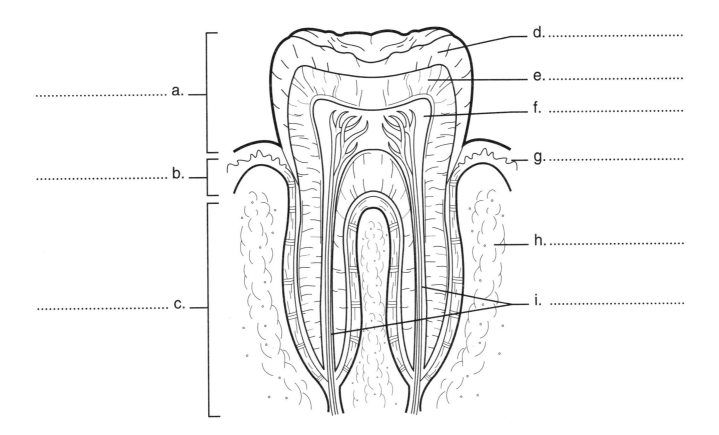

.... a.

.... b.

.... c.

d. ....

e. ....

f. ....

g. ....

h. ....

i. ....

FIGURE **9–1** BASIC STRUCTURE AND CIRCULATION OF THE HEART
The figure below illustrates the basic structure and circulation of the heart. Identify the structures that are labeled with a blank line, and color each structure a different color.

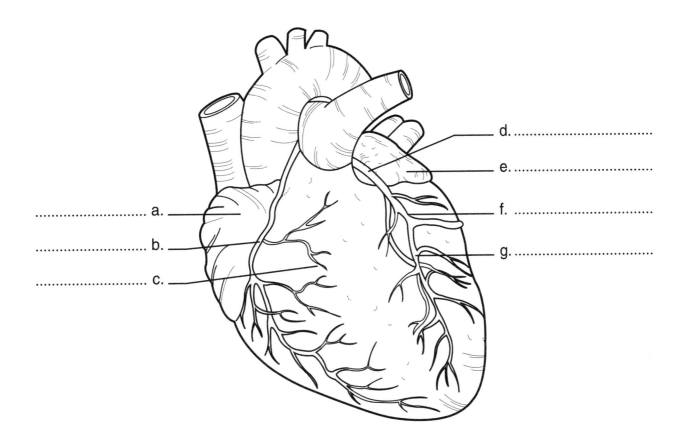

d. ....

e. ....

.... a. ——————

f. ....

.... b. ——————

g. ....

.... c. ——————

FIGURE **9–2** **CROSS-SECTION OF THE HEART**
The figure below illustrates a cross-section of the heart. Identify the structures that are labeled with a blank line and color each identified structure a different color.

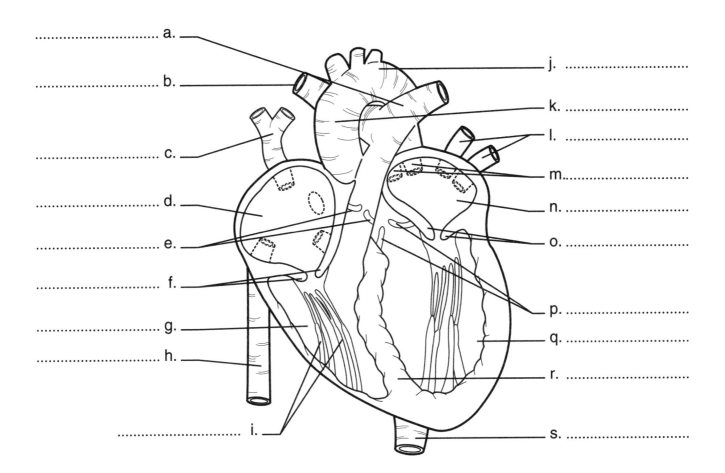

.... a.

.... b.

.... c.

.... d.

.... e.

.... f.

.... g.

.... h.

.... i.

j. ....

k. ....

l. ....

m............................

n. ....

o. ....

p. ....

q. ....

r. ....

s. ....

FIGURE **9–3** **HOW THE HEART BEATS**
The figure below illustrates the heartbeat sequence. Identify the sequence by filling in the blank under the picture.

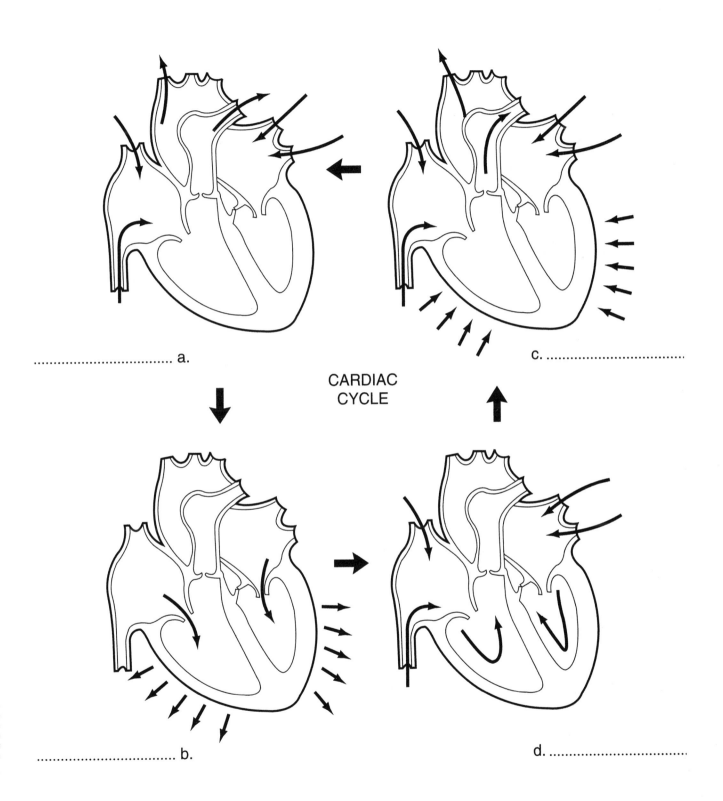

.... a.

CARDIAC
CYCLE

c. ....

.... b.

d. ....

UNIT 10 The Circulatory System

FIGURE **10-1** TYPES OF BLOOD VESSELS (Arterioles)
The figure below illustrates a cross-section of a closed system of blood vessels to the four chamber of the heart. Blood travels away from the heart through arteries, which branch into smaller vessels, the arterioles. Identify the structures, which are labeled with a blank line, and color each structure with a different color.

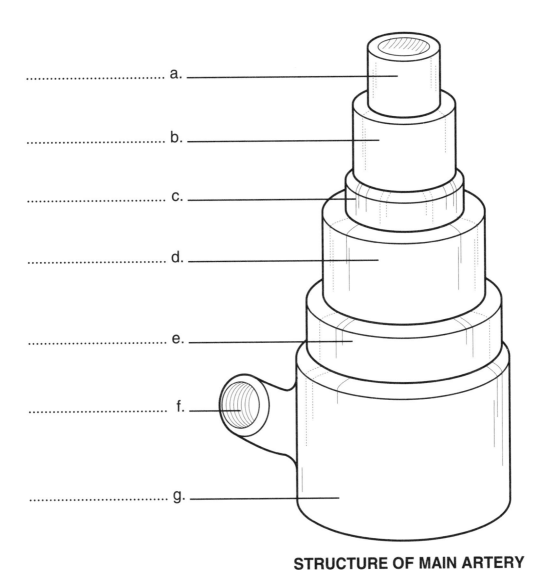

.... a.

.... b.

.... c.

.... d.

.... e.

.... f.

.... g.

STRUCTURE OF MAIN ARTERY

FIGURE **10–2** TYPES OF BLOOD VESSELS (Venous)
The figure below illustrates a cross-section of a closed system of blood vessels to and from the four chambers of the heart. Blood travels or returns to the heart as capillaries merge to form venules, which further merge to form larger veins, which connect to the heart. Identify the structures, which are labeled with a blank line, and color each structure with a different color.

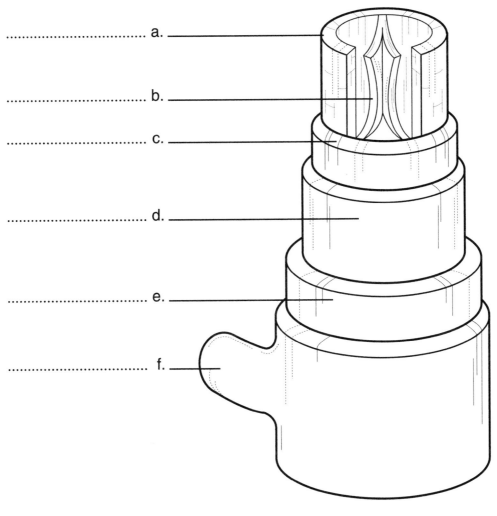

.... a.

.... b.

.... c.

.... d.

.... e.

.... f.

STRUCTURE OF MAIN VEIN

UNIT 10 The Circulatory System

FIGURE **10–3** HOW THE SYSTEM WORKS (Arterioles)
The figure below illustrates a cross-section of the arterial vessels of the body including the four chambers of the heart. Identify the structures, which are labeled with a blank line, and color each structure with a different color.

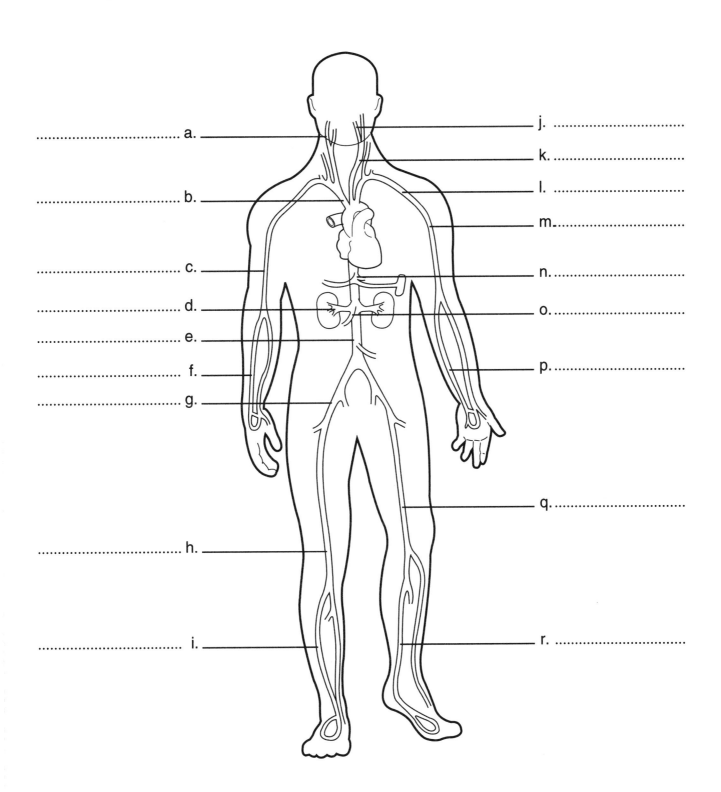

.... a.

.... b.

.... c.

.... d.

.... e.

.... f.

.... g.

.... h.

.... i.

j. ....

k. ....

l. ....

m...............................

n. ....

o. ....

p. ....

q. ....

r. ....

UNIT 10 The Circulatory System

FIGURE **10–4** HOW THE SYSTEM WORKS (Venous)
The figure below illustrates a cross-section of the veins of the body. Identify the structures, which are labeled with a blank line, and color each structure with a different color.

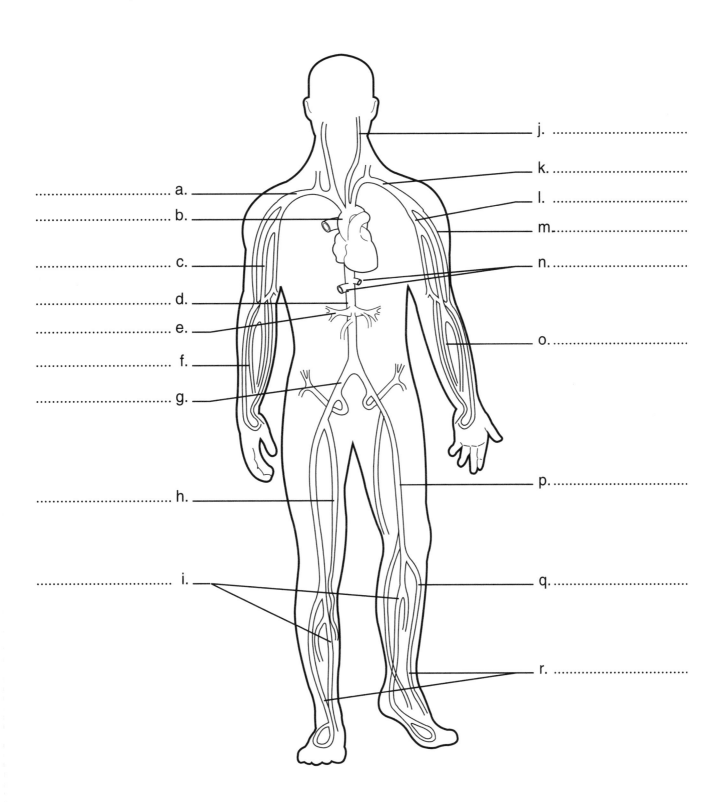

a. ....

b. ....

c. ....

d. ....

e. ....

f. ....

g. ....

h. ....

i. ....

j. ....

k. ....

l. ....

m. ....

n. ....

o. ....

p. ....

q. ....

r. ....

UNIT 11 The Lungs

FIGURE **11–1** BASIC LUNG STRUCTURES

The figure below pictures the lungs, bronchial tree, lobes of the lungs, and a cross-section view. Carefully identify all areas that are indicated with lines, and remember that spelling accuracy is important. Once identified, color the specific structures using a different color for each section.

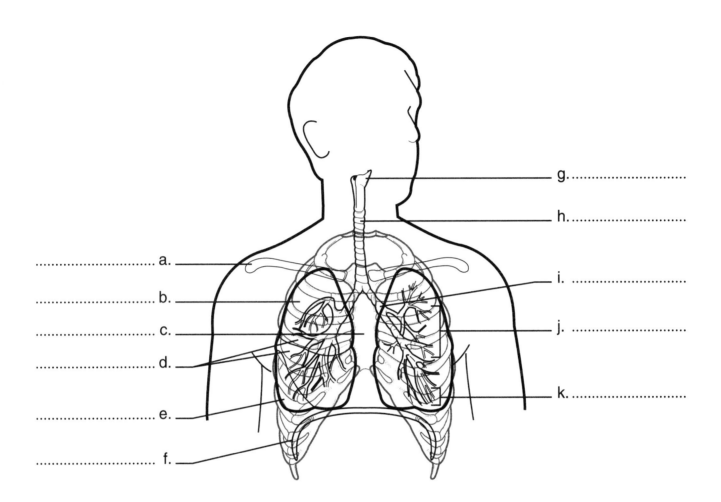

UNIT 12 The Lymphatic System and Spleen

FIGURE 12–1 (Overview)   THE LYMPHATIC SYSTEM AND SPLEEN
The figure below illustrates the lymphatic system, which is a series of vessels, structures, and organs that collect fluid throughout the body and return it to the main circulation for redistribution. The system also contains cells called lymphocytes (white blood cells) that help fight infection. Identify each structure labeled with a blank line, and color each structure a different color. All lymph nodes, regardless of their location, can be colored the same color.

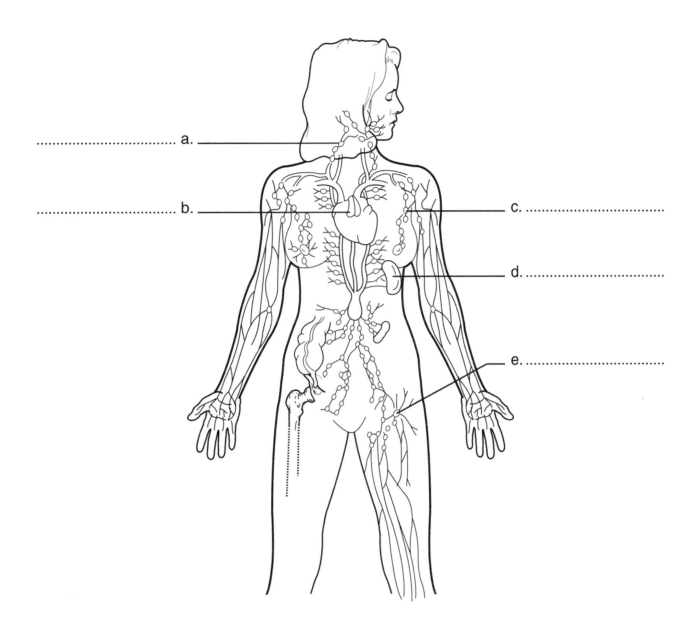

.... a.

.... b.

c. ....

d. ....

e. ....

UNIT 13 The Endocrine System

FIGURE **13-1** TYPES OF ENDOCRINE GLANDS
The figure below is an illustration of the various endocrine glands of the body. These glands secrete hormones into the bloodstream that travel throughout the body. These secretions affect organs as well as other endocrine glands to control specific actions within the body. Identify each gland indicated by the blank lines. Color each structure a different color.

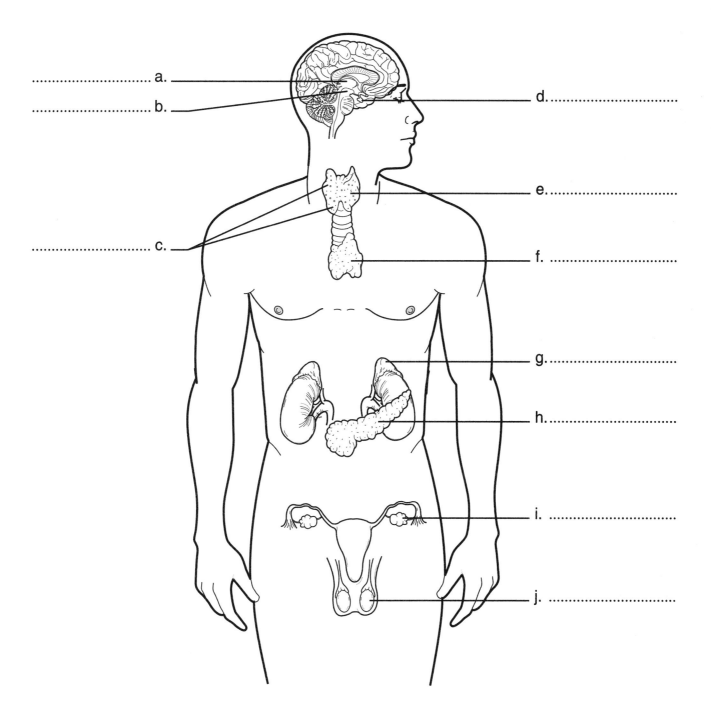

.... a. _____

.... b. _____

d. ....

e. ....

.... c. _____

f. ....

g. ....

h. ....

i. ....

j. ....

FIGURE **14–1** BASIC DIGESTIVE SYSTEM STRUCTURE

The digestive system processes food so that it can be absorbed and used by the body's cells. The structures identified below are responsible for food ingestion, digestion, absorption, and elimination of undigested remains from the body. Select different colors for the organs identified by the blank lines. Color the structures and fill in the blanks with the correct names.

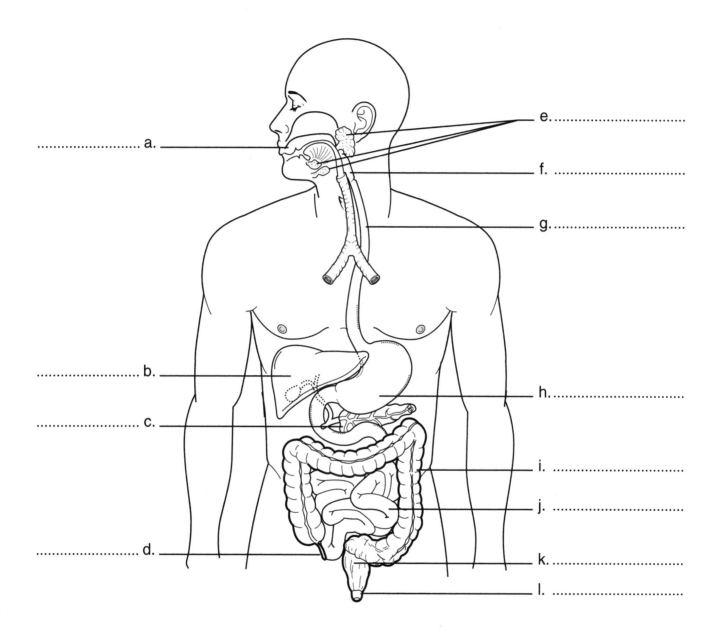

.... a. ____

.... b. ____

.... c. ____

.... d. ____

e. ....

f. ....

g. ....

h. ....

i. ....

j. ....

k. ....

l. ....

UNIT 14 The Digestive System

FIGURE **14–2** **STOMACH (Cross-section)**
The structure identified below is a cross-section of the stomach. The stomach is a large sac that begins to digest the proteins in food. When the food is digested, it is converted into chemicals that the body can use for energy, growth, and repair. Identify the various sections of the stomach by filling in the blank lines, and color each section a different color.

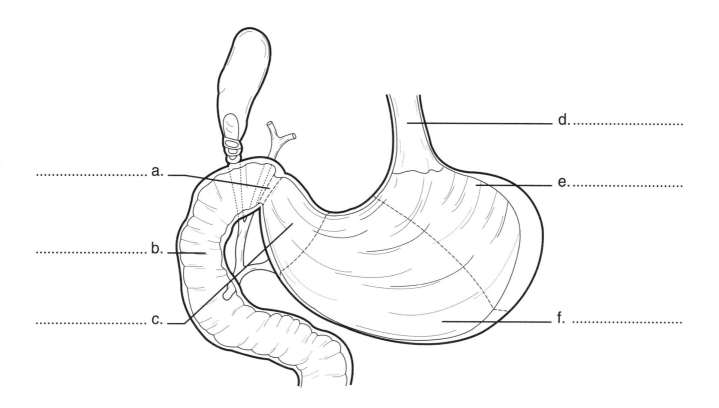

UNIT 14   The Digestive System

FIGURE **14–3**   SMALL AND LARGE INTESTINES (Cross-section)
The structure identified below is a cross-section of the small and large intestines. From the stomach, food passes through several parts of the small intestine, where digestion is completed and food nutrients are absorbed into the blood. In the large intestine, the stool absorbs water and becomes more solid waste, waiting to be eliminated from the body. Identify each section by filling in the blank lines, and color each structure a different color.

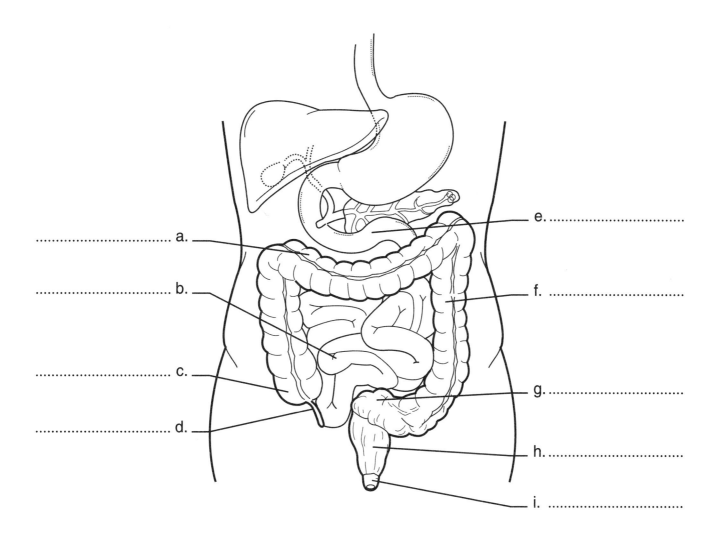

.... a.

.... b.

.... c.

.... d.

e. ....

f. ....

g. ....

h. ....

i. ....

UNIT 15 The Urinary System

FIGURE **15–1** BASIC URINARY SYSTEM STRUCTURE

The urinary system eliminates liquid wastes from the body. Each of the body's cells discharge wastes into the bloodstream, which carries these wastes to the kidneys located on either side of the spine in the lumbar region. The picture below illustrates the entire urinary system: kidneys, ureters, bladder, and urethra. Fill in the blank lines and color each structure identified.

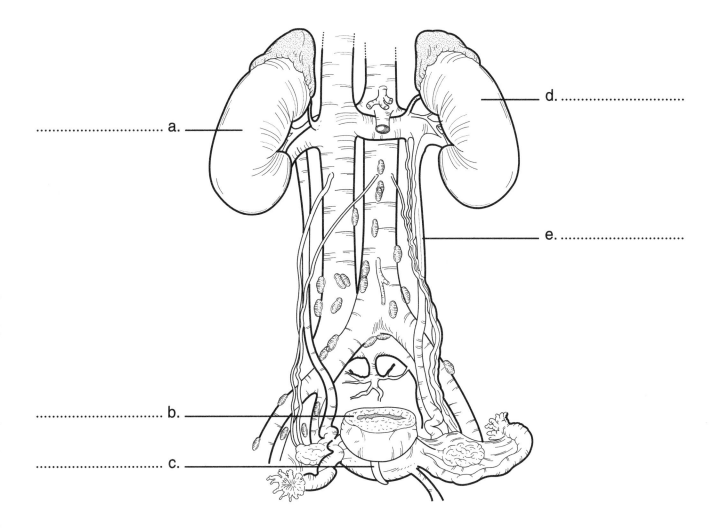

a. ....

b. ....

c. ....

d. ....

e. ....

FIGURE **15–2**   **CROSS-SECTION OF THE KIDNEY**

The kidneys filter wastes from the bloodstream. The waste products enter the kidneys via the renal artery, and some are returned to the circulation by way of the renal vein. Other by-products are filtered through and excreted through the renal pelvis to the ureters. Identify the structures below and fill in the blank lines. Color each structure identified a different color.

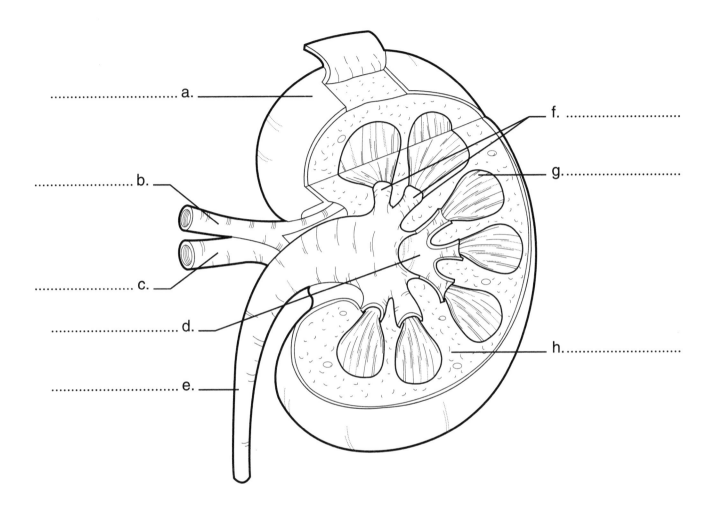

UNIT 16 Male Reproductive System

FIGURE **16–1** BASIC STRUCTURE
The structure identified below is a cross-section of the male reproductive system, including the testes and the urogenital structure. Fill in the structures that are identified with a blank line, and color each structure to be identified with a different color.

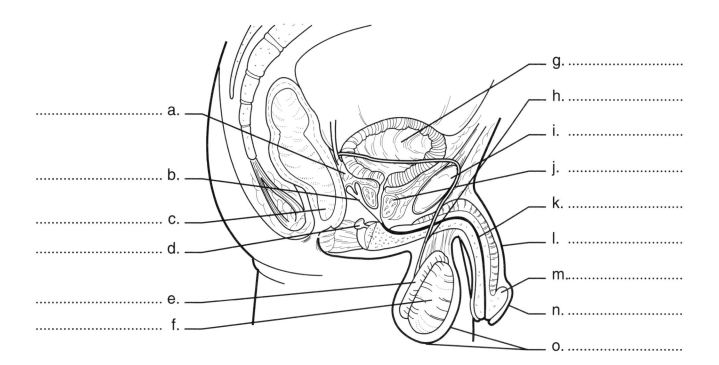

.... a.

.... b.

.... c.

.... d.

.... e.

.... f.

g. ....

h. ....

i. ....

j. ....

k. ....

l. ....

m. ....

n. ....

o. ....

UNIT 17 Female Reproductive System

FIGURE **17-1 BASIC STRUCTURE (Cross-section or ventral view)**
The figure below illustrates the cross-section or ventral view of the female reproductive system. The organs of the reproductive system create human offspring by combining genes from a man and a woman. The female reproductive organs help to develop and nurture the fetus. Each structure is identified by a blank line. Fill in the blank lines and color each structure a different color.

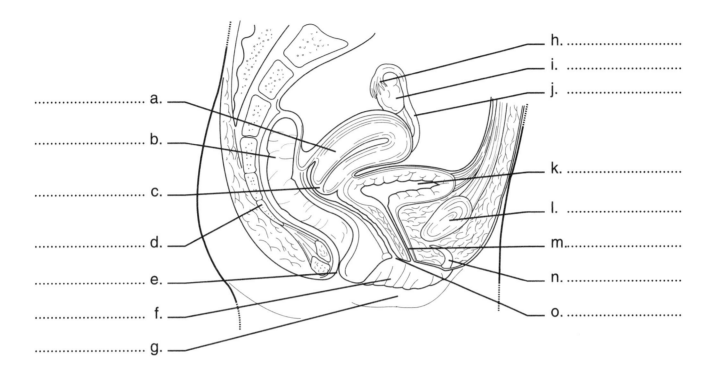

.... a.

.... b.

.... c.

.... d.

.... e.

.... f.

.... g.

h. ....

i. ....

j. ....

k. ....

l. ....

m. ....

n. ....

o. ....

UNIT 17 Female Reproductive System

FIGURE **17–2** POSTERIOR VIEW
The figure below illustrates a posterior view of the female reproductive system. This structure is located in the pelvic portion of the abdominopelvic cavity. Fill in the blanks of each structure indicated and color each structure a different color.

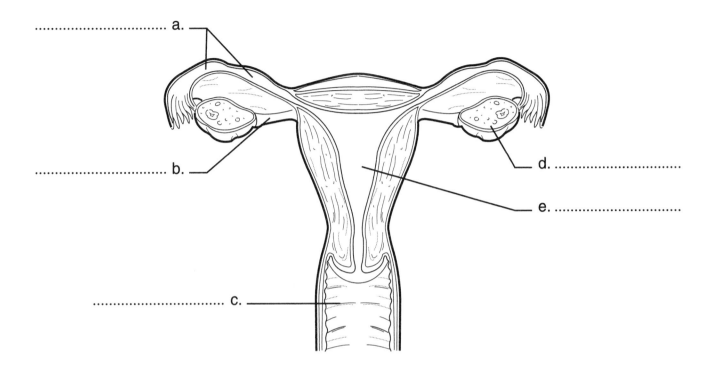

113

UNIT 17 Female Reproductive System

FIGURE 17–3 EXTERNAL GENITALIA
The figure below illustrates a view of the external female genitalia, a diamond-shaped area medial to the thighs and buttocks also known as the perineum. This is known as the external reproductive structure of the body. Identify the structures marked with a blank line and color them with a different color.

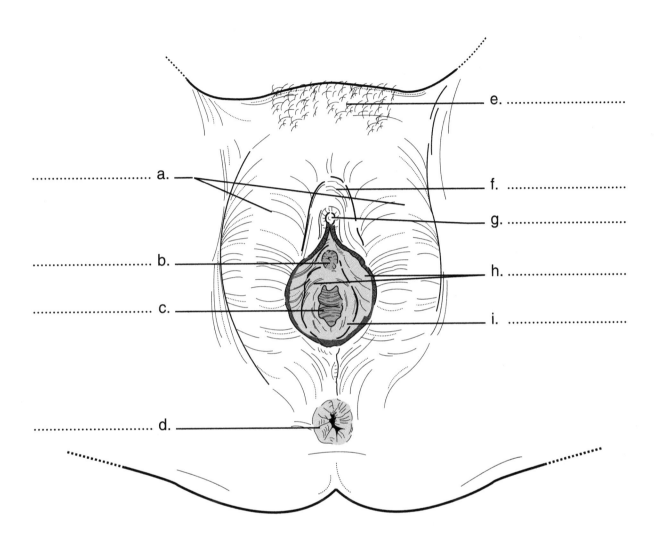

FIGURE **17–4** BREAST (Cross-section)

The figure below illustrates a cross-section view of the breast. The female breast contains mammary glands, which are modified sweat glands that produce and secrete milk for human offspring. Review the structures associated with these glands and identify the structures indicated with a blank line. Color each structure a different color.

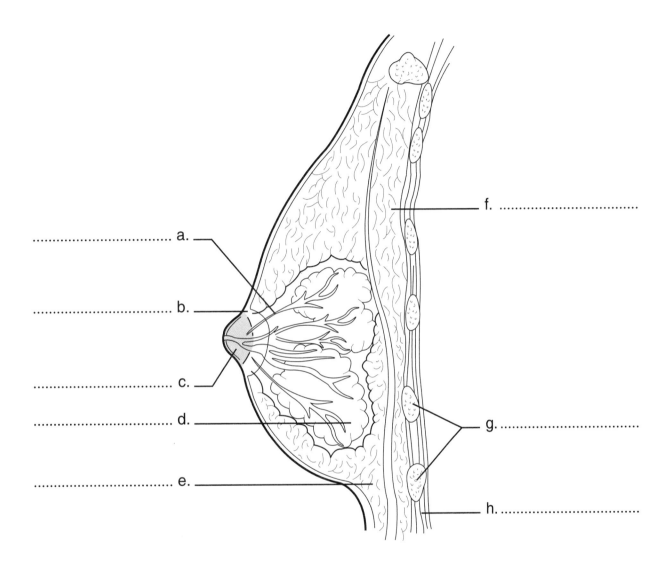

PRONUNCIATION GUIDE

NOTE: In the pronunciations given below, the prime symbol (′) indicates which syllable is stressed in the word; in words with more than one stressed syllable, the syllable with secondary stress is indicated by a double prime symbol (″). Vowels are pronounced as follows: ā as in day; a as in bat; ă as in about; ē as in be; ĕ as in met; ī as in pine; ĭ as in pit; ō as in no; ŏ as in got; oy as in boy; ū as in food; ŭ as in but; and yū as in unit.

-A-

abducens – ab-dū′senz
accessory – ak-ses′ō-rē
acetabulum – as″ĕ-tab′yū-lŭm
adipose tissue – ad′i-pōs tish′ū
adrenal gland – ă-drē′năl gland
alveolar bone – al-vē′ō-lăr bōn
amphiarthrosis – am″fi-ar-thrō′sis
anterior canal – an-tēr′ē-ōr kă-nal′
anterior cardiac vein – an-tēr′ē-ōr kar′dē-ak vān
anterior tibial – an-tēr′ē-ōr tib′ē-ăl
anus – ā′nŭs
aorta – ā-ōr′tă
aortic arch – ā-ōr′tik arch
aortic semilunar valve – ā-ōr′tik sem″ē-lū′năr valv
apex – ā′peks
appendix – ă-pen′diks
arachnoid – ă-rak′noyd
arachnoid villus – ă-rak′noyd vil′ŭs
areola – ă-rē′ō-lă
arrector pili – ă-rek′tōr pī′lī
arteriole – ar-tēr′ē-ōl
articular cartilage – ar-tik′yu-lăr kar′ti-lij
atlas – at′las
auditory canal – aw′di-tōr″ē kă-nal′
axillary – ak′sil-ār-ē
axon – ak′son

-B-

biceps – bī′seps
bicuspid – bī-kŭs′pid
bladder – blad′er
brachial – brā′kē-ăl
brachialis – brā″kē-ā′lis
brachial plexus – brā′kē-ăl plek′sŭs
brachiocephalic – brăk′ē-ō-se-fal′ik
brachioradialis – brăk″ē-ō-rā″dē-ā′līs
brachycephalic – brak′ē-se-fal′ik
brain stem – brān stem
bulbourethral gland – bŭl″bō-yū-rē′thrăl gland

-C-

calcaneal tendon – kal-kā′nē-al ten′dŏn
calcaneus – kal-kā′nē-ŭs
calyx – kā′liks
canine – kā′nīn
cardiac muscle – kar′dē-ak mŭs′ĕl
carpal – kar′păl
cecum – sē′kŭm
celiac trunk – sē′lē-ak trŭnk
cell body – sel bod′ē
central canal – sen′trăl kă-nal′
cephalic – se-fal′ik
cerebellum – ser-e-bel′ŭm
cerebral cortex – ser′ĕ-brăl kōr′teks

cerebral hemisphere – ser′ĕ-brăl hem′i-sfēr
cerebrum – ser′ĕ-brŭm
cervical – ser′-vĭ-kal
cervical vertebrae – ser′-vĭ-kal ver′tĕ-brā
cervix – ser′viks
choroid – ko′-royd
ciliary body – sil′ĕ-ar″ē bod′ē
ciliary muscle – sil′ĕ-ar″ē mŭs′ĕl
circumflex – ser′kŭm-fleks
clavicle – klav′i-kl
clitoris – klit′ō-ris
coccyx, fused – kok′siks, fyūzd
cochlea – kok′lē-ă
collagen – kol′ă-jen
common iliac – kom′min il′ē-ak
compact bone – kom′pakt bōn
condyloid joint – kon′di-loyd joynt
conjunctiva – kon″jŭnk-tī′vă
cornea – kōr′nē-ă
cortex – kōr′teks
costal cartilage – kos′tăl kar′ti-lij
cranial nerve – krā′nē-ăl nerv
cricoid cartilage – krī′koyd kar′ti-lij
cricothyroid ligament – krī-kō-thī′royd lig′ă-ment
crown – krown
cuspid – kŭs′pid

-D-

deltoid – del′toyd
dendrite – den′drīt
dentin – den′tin
dermis – der′mis
diaphragm – dī′ă-fram
diaphysis – dī-af′i-sis
diarthrosis – dī-ar-thrō′sis
distal epiphysis – dis′tăl e-pif′i-sis
distal phalanx – dis′tăl fa′langks
dorsal root – dōr′săl rūt
ductus deferens – dŭk′tŭs def′ĕr-enz
duodenum – dū″ō-dē′nŭm
dural sinus – dū′răl sī′nŭs
dura mater – dū′ră mā′ter

-E-

eardrum – ēr′drŭm
ejaculatory duct – ē-jak′yū-lă-tōr″-ē dŭkt
elastic fiber – ĕ-las′tik fī′ber
endosteum – en-dos′tē-ŭm
endothelium – ĕn″dō-thē′lē-ŭm
epidermis – ep″i-der′mis
epididymis – ep″i-did′i-mis
epiglottis – ep″i-glot′is
esophagus – ē-sof′ă-gŭs
ethmoid bone – eth′moyd bōn
Eustachian tube – yū-stā′kē-ăn tūb

excretion – eks-krē'shŭn
external carotid – eks-ter'năl ka-rot'id
external elastic lamina – eks-ter'năl ĕ-las'tik lam'i-nă
external oblique – eks-ter'năl ob-lēk'

-F-

facial – fā'shăl
fallopian tube – fa-lō'pē-an tūb
false rib – fawls rib
falx cerebri – falks ser'e-brī
fat or adipose tissue – fat/ad'i-pōs tish'ū
femoral – fem'ŏ-răl
femur – fē'mŭr
fibula – fib'yū-lă
fibular notch – fib'yū-lăr notch
flat bone – flat bōn
flexor carpi radialis – flek'sōr kar'pī rā"dē-ā'lis
flexor carpi ulnaris – flek'sōr kar'pī ŭl-nā'ris
floating rib – flōt-ing rib
foramen magnum – fō-rā'men mag'nŭm
fovea centralis – fō've-ă sen-trā'lis
frontal bone – frŭn'tăl bōn
frontalis – frŭn'tā'lis
frontal lobe – frŭn'tăl lōb
fundus – fŭn'dŭs

-G-

gastrocnemius – gas"trok-nē'mē-ŭs
gingival – jin'ji-văl
greater saphenous – grāt'er să-fē'nŭs
greater trochanter – grāt'er trō-kan'ter

-H-

hard palate –-hard pal'ăt
head of fibula – hed of fib'yū-lă
helix – hē'liks
hepatic – he-pat'ik
humerus – hyū'mer-ŭs
hyoid bone – hī'oyd bōn
hypoglossal – hī"pō-glos'ăl
hypothalamus – hī"pō-thal'ă-mŭs

-I-

ileum – il'ē-ŭm
iliac crest – il'ē-ak krest
iliac fossa – il'ē-ăk fos'ă
iliac lymph node – il'ē-ak limf nōd
incisors – in-sī'zŏr
index finger – in'deks fing'ger'
inferior lobe – in-fē'rē-ōr lōb
inferior vena cava – in-fē'rē-ōr vē'nă cā'vă
inner ear – i'nĕr ēr
inner layer – i'ner lā'er
intact lung – in-takt' lŭng
intercostal muscle – in"ter-kos'tăl mŭs'ĕl
intercostal space – in"ter-kos'tăl spās
internal elastic lamina – in-ter'năl ĕ-las'tik lam'i-nă
internal jugular – in-ter'năl jŭg'yū-lar
internal oblique – in-ter'năl ob-lēk'
interosseus membrane – in"ter-ōs'ē-ŭs mem'brăn
intraventricular septum – in"tră-ven-trik'yū-lăr sep'tŭm
iris – ī'ris
ischium – is'kē-ŭm

-L-

labia majora – lā'bē-ă mā-jo'ră
labia minora – lā'bē-ă mī-no'ră
lacrimal bone – lak'ri-măl bōn
large intestine – lărj in-tes'tin
larynx – lar'ingks
lateral condyle of tibia – lat'er-ăl kon'dīl of tib'ē-ă
lateral epicondyle of femur – lat'er-ăl ep"i-kon'dīl of fē'mŭr
lateral malleolus – lat'er-ăl ma-lē'ō-lŭs
latissimus dorsi – la-tis'i-mŭs dōr'sī
left atrium – left ā'trē-ŭm
left auricle – left aw'ri-kl
left AV valve – left AV valv
left coronary artery – left kōr'o-nā-rē ar'ter-ē
left kidney – left kid'nē
left pulmonary artery – left pŭl'mō-nā-rē ar'ter-ē
left pulmonary vein – left pŭl'mō-nā-rē vān
left ventricle – left ven'tri-kl
lens – lenz
lesser trochanter – le'ser trō-kan'ter
little finger – li'tel fing'ger
lingual tonsil – lĭng'gwăl ton'sil
liver – liv'er
long bone – long bōn
lumbar – lŭm'bar
lumbar vertebrae – lŭm'bar ver'tĕ-brā

-M-

macula – mak'yū-lă
mammary duct – mam'ă-rē dŭkt
mammary gland – mam'ă-rē gland
mandible – man'di-bl
mandibular fossa – man-dib'yū-lăr fos'ă
manubrium – mă-nū'brē-ŭm
maxilla – mak'sil-ă
medial condyle of tibia – mē'dē-ăl kon'dīl of tib'ē-ă
medial epicondyle of femur – mē'dē-ăl ep"i-kon'dīl of fē'mŭr
medial malleolus – mē'dē-ăl ma-lē'ō-lŭs
mediastinum – me"dē-as-tī'nŭm
medulla oblongata – me-dūl'ă ob"long-gah'tă
medullary cavity – mē'dul'er-ē kav'i-tē
metabolism – mĕ-tab'ō-lizm
metacarpals – met'ă-kar-păl
metaphysis – me-taf'i-sis
metatarsal – met'ă-tar'săl
middle finger – mid'l fing'ger
molar – mō'lăr
mons pubis – monz pyū'bis
myelin sheath – mī'ĕ-lin shēth

-N-

nasal bone – nā'zăl bōn
nasal cavity – nā'zăl kav'i-tē
nerve fiber – nerv fī'ber
neurilemma – nūr'ī-lem'ă
nipple – nip'l
node of Ranvier – nōd of răn-vē-ā'
nucleus – nū'klē-ŭs

-O-

obturator foramen – ob'tū-rā"tŏr fō-rā'men
occipital bone – ok-sip'i-tăl bōn

occipitalis – ok″sip-i-tā′lis
occipital lobe – ok-sip′i-tăl lōb
oculomotor – ok″yū-lō-mō′tŏr
olfactory – ol-fak′tŏ-rē
optic – op′tik
optic nerve – op′tik nerv
orbicularis oculi – ōr-bik″yū-lā′ris ok′yū-lī
orbicularis oris – ōr-bik″yū-lā′ris ōr′is
organ of Corti – ōr′găn of kōr′tī
oval window – ō′val win′dō
ovarian fimbriae – ō-vār′ē-an fim′brē-ā
ovarian ligament – ō-vār′ē-an lĭg′ă-mĕnt
ovary – ō′vă-rē

-P-

palatine tonsil – pal′ă-tīn ton′sil
palmaris longus – pawl-mār′is long′ŭs
pancreas – pan′krē-as
papilla – pă-pil′ă
papillae – pă-pil′ă
papillary muscle – păp′i-lār-ē mŭs′ĕl
parathyroid gland – par-ă-thī′royd gland
parietal bone – pă-rī′ĕ-tăl bōn
parietal lobe – pă-rī′ĕ-tăl lōb
patella – pa-tel′ă
pectoralis major – pek″tō-ral′is mā′jŏr
periosteum – per″-ē-os′tē-ŭm
phalanges – fă-lan′jēz
pharynx – far′ĭngks
pia mater – pē′ă mā′ter
pineal gland – pin′ē-ăl gland
pituitary gland – pi-tū′i-tār″ē gland
pivot joint – piv′ŏt joynt
plantaris – plan-tār′is
pons – ponz
popliteal – pop″li-tē′ăl
posterior canal – pos-tēr′ē-ŏr kă-nal′
posterior tibial – pos-tēr′ē-ŏr tib′ē-ăl
premolar – prē-mō′lăr
prepuce – prē′pūs
primary bronchus – prī′mar-ē brong′kŭs
pronator teres – prō-nā′tōr ter′ēz
proximal phalanx – prok′si-măl fa′langks
pubic symphysis – pyū′bik sim′fi-sis
pubis – pyū′bis
pulmonary semilunar valve – pŭl′mō-nā-rē sem″ē-lū′năr valv
pulp cavity – pŭlp kav′i-tē
pupil – pyū′pĭl
pyloric sphincter – pī-lōr′ik sfingk′ter
pylorus – pī-lōr′ŭs

-R-

radial – rā′dē-ăl
radius – rā′dē-ŭs
rectum – rek′tŭm
renal – rē′năl
renal artery – rē′năl ar′ter-ē
renal column – rē′năl kol′ŭm
renal pelvis – rē′năl pel′vis
renal pyramid – rē′năl pir′ă-mid
renal vein – rē′năl vān
retina – ret′i-nă

retinal blood vessel – ret′i-năl blŭd ves′ĕl
rib – rib
right atrium – rīt ā′trē-ŭm
right AV valve – rīt AV valv
right coronary artery – rīt kōr′o-nā-rē ar′ter-ē
right pulmonary artery – rīt pŭl′mō-nā-rē ar′ter-ē pŭl-mō-nĕ-rē ăr′tĕr-ē
right pulmonary vein – rīt pŭl′mō-nā-rē vān
right ventricle – rīt ven′tri-kl
root – rūt
root canal – rūt kă-nal′

-S-

sacral promontory – sā′krăl prom′on-tō″rē
sacral vertebrae – sā′krăl ver′tĕ-brā
sacrum – sā′krŭm
salivary gland – sal′i-vār-ē gland
scalp – skalp
scapula – skap′yū-lă
sclera – sklēr′ă
Schwann cell nucleus – shvŏn sel nū′klē-ŭs
sebaceous gland – sē-bā′shŭs gland
secondary bronchus – sek′ŏn-dār-ē brong′kŭs
semicircular canal – sem″ē-sir′kyū-lăr kă-nal′
seminal vesicle – sem′i-năl ves′i-kl
sensation – sen-sā′shŭn
sesamoid bone – ses′ă-moyd bōn
short bone – short bōn
sigmoid colon – sig′moyd kō′lon
skeletal muscle – skel′ĕ-tăl mŭs′ĕl
skull bone – skŭl bōn
small intestine – smawl′ in-tes′tin
soft palate – soft pal′ăt
soleus – sō′lē-ŭs
sphenoid bone – sfē′noyd bōn
sphenoid process – sfē′noyd pros′es
spleen – splēn
sternocleidomastoid – ster″nō-klī″dō-mas′toyd
sternum – ster′nŭm
stomach – stŭm′ŭk
stratum basale – strā′tŭm bā-sa′l
stratum corneum – strā′tŭm kōr′nē-ŭm
subarachnoid space – sŭb″ă-rak′noyd spās
subclavian – sŭb-klā′vē-an
subcutaneous – sŭb″kyū-tā′nē-ŭs
sweat – swet
sweat gland – swet gland
symphysis – sim′fi-sis
synarthrosis – sin″ar-thrō′sis

-T-

tarsal – tar′săl
temporal bone – tem′pŏ-răl bōn
temporalis – tem-pŏ-rā′lis
temporal lobe – tem′pŏ-răl lōb
terminal branches – ter′mi-năl branch-ĕz
tertiary bronchus – ter′shē-ăr-ē brong′kŭs
testes – tes′tēz
testis – tes′tis
thoracic – thō-ras′ik
thoracic vertebrae – thō-ras′ik ver′tĕ-brā
thymus gland – thī′mŭs gland
thyrohyoid membrane – thī″rō-hī′oyd mem′brān

thyroid cartilage – thī'royd kar'ti-lij
thyroid gland – thī'royd gland
tibia – tib'ē-ă
tongue – tŭng
trachea – trā'kē-ă
tracheal cartilage – trā'kē-ăl kar'ti-lij
transverse colon – tran-vers' kō'lon
trapezius – tra-pē'zē-ŭs
triceps – trī'seps
trigeminal – trī-jem'i-năl
trochlear – trok'lē-ar
true rib – trū rib
tunicae media – tū'ni-kā mē'dē-ă

-U-

ulna – ŭl'nă
ureter – yū'rē-ter
urethra – yū-rē'thră
urethral orifice – yū-rē'thrăl or'i-fis
urinary bladder – yūr'i-nār''ē blad'er
uterine tube – yū'ter-in tūb
uterus – yū'ter-ŭs

-V-

vagina – vă-jī'nă
vaginal orifice – vaj'i-năl or'i-fis

vagus – vā'gŭs
valve cusp – valv kŭsp
ventral root – ven'trăl rūt
ventricular systole – ven-trik'yū-lăr [vĕn-trĭk'ū-lăr] sis'tō-lē
vertebral bone – ver'tĕ-brăl bōn
vestibule – ves'ti-būl
vestibulocochlear – ves-tib''yū-lō-kok'lē-ăr
vitreous body – vit'rē-ŭs bod'ē
vocal cord – vō'kăl kōrd
vomer bone – vō'mer bōn

-W-

white matter – hwīt ma'ter

-X-

xiphoid process – zif'oyd pros'es

-Z-

zygomatic facial foramen – zī''gō-mat'ik fā'shăl fō-rā'men
zygomaticus – zī''gō-mat'ik-ŭs

ANSWER KEY

UNIT 1 The Skin

FIG. **1-1** Layers of the skin
a. epidermis
b. dermis
c. subcutaneous (fatty tissue)

FIG. **1-2** Accessory organs of the skin
a. hair shaft
b. stratum corneum
c. stratum germinativum
d. sebaceous gland
e. arrector pili muscle
f. nerve fibers
g. sweat gland
h. hair follicle
i. fat or adipose tissue

UNIT 2 The Skeletal System

FIG. **2-1** Types of bones
a. flat bone
b. irregular bone
c. long bone
d. sesamoid bone
e. short bone

FIG. **2-2** Bone structure
a. proximal epiphysis
b. metaphysis
c. diaphysis
d. metaphysis
e. distal epiphysis
f. red marrow (spongy bone)
g. compact bone
h. medullary cavity
i. yellow marrow
j. periosteum
k. condyles

FIG. **2-3** Skull (lateral view)
a. frontal bone
b. zygomatic bone
c. parietal bone
d. temporal bone
e. occipital bone

FIG. **2-4** Cranium (inferior view)
a. sphenoid process
b. mastoid process
c. zygomatic process
d. zygomatic bone
e. foramen magnum
f. mandibular fossa
g. maxilla

FIG. **2-5** Facial bones
a. temporal bone
b. ethmoid bone
c. nasal bone
d. zygomatic bone
e. maxilla
f. mandible
g. frontal bone
h. maxilla
i. sphenoid bone
j. ethmoid bone
k. vomer bone

FIG. **2-6** Vertebral sections (cervical, thoracic, lumbar, sacral)
a. atlas C1
b. axis C2
c. cervical
d. thoracic
e. lumbar
f. sacrum fused
g. coccyx fused

FIG. **2-7** Vertebral sections (various types)
a. atlas
b. cervical
c. thoracic
d. lumbar

FIG. **2-8** Thorax (sternum, ribs and false ribs, and cartilage)
a. manubrium
b. sternum body
c. xiphoid process
d. costal cartilage
e. intercostal space
f. floating rib
g. true ribs
h. false ribs

FIG. **2-9** Pectoral girdle (upper extremity, clavicle, scapula)
a. clavicle
b. radius
c. costal cartilage
d. scapula
e. humerus
f. ulna

Pectoral girdle (hand)
FIG. **2-10** Anterior view
a. radius
b. carpals
c. metacarpals

FIG. **2-11** Posterior view
a. ulna
b. metacarpals
c. little finger
d. ring finger
e. middle finger

Answer Key

f. radius
g. carpals
h. proximal phalanx
i. distal phalanx
j. phalanges
k. index finger

FIG. **2-12**   Pelvic girdle

a. sacral promontory
b. sacrum
c. coccyx
d. pubic symphysis
e. pubic arch
f. iliac crest
g. iliac fossa
h. pubis (pubic bone)
i. acetabulum
j. oburator foramen
k. ischium

Lower limbs (Bones of the lower limbs)
FIG. **2-13**   Anterior view

a. lateral condyle of tibia
b. head of fibula
c. fibula
d. interosseus membrane
e. fibular notch
f. lateral malleolus
g. medial condyle of tibia
h. lateral condyle of tibia
i. head of fibula
j. fibula
k. tibia
l. interosseus membrane
m. medial malleolus

Lower limbs (bones of the leg)
FIG. **2-14**   Anterior view

a. greater trochanter
b. patella
c. tibia
d. fibula
e. lateral malleolus
f. lesser trochanter
g. femur

FIG. **2-15**   Posterior view

a. head of femur
b. neck of femur
c. lesser trochanter
d. body of femur
e. tibia
f. greater trochanter
g. femur
h. fibula

FIG. **2-16**   Bones of the foot

a. tarsals
b. metatarsals
c. phalanges
d. tibia
e. calcaneus

FIG. **2-17**   Structures of the knee

a. femur
b. patella
c. lateral epicondyle of femur
d. tibia
e. fibula
f. medial epicondyle of femur

FIG. **2-18**   Joints

a. amphiathrosis (slightly movable joint), cartilaginous joint
b. synarthrois (immovable joint), fibrous joint
c. diathrosis (freely movable joint), synovial
d. condyloid joint
e. ball & socket joint
f. gliding joint
g. saddle joint
h. hinge joint
i. pivot joint

UNIT 3   The Muscular System

FIG. **3-1**   Types of muscles

a. cardiac muscle
b. skeletal muscle
c. smooth muscle

FIG. **3-2**   Skeletal muscles of the head

a. temporalis
b. frontalis
c. obicularis oculi
d. zygomaticus
e. orbicularis oris
f. sternocleidomastoid
g. occipitalis
h. trapezius

FIG. **3-3**   Muscles of the trunk (anterior view)

a. trapezius
b. pectoralis major
c. biceps
d. external oblique
e. sternocleidomastoid
f. sternum
g. rectus abdominis

FIG. **3-4**   Muscles of the trunk (posterior view)

a. trapezius
b. latissimus dorsi
c. sternocleidomastoid
d. deltoid

e. triceps
f. external oblique

FIG. **3-5** Muscles of the arm & forearm
a. deltoid
b. pectoralis major
c. triceps
d. biceps
e. brachialis
f. pronator teres
g. brachioradalis
h. flexor carpi radialis
i. palmaris longus
j. flexor carpi ulnaris

FIG. **3-6** Muscles of the hip, thigh, and leg
a. soleus
b. gastrocnemius
c. biceps femoris
d. calcaneal tendon

UNIT 4 The Nervous System

FIG. **4-1** Basic neuron
a. cell body
b. nucleus
c. dendrites
d. axon
e. axonal terminals
f. myelin sheath
g. neurilemma
h. node of ranvier
i. schwann cell nucleus

FIG. **4-2** Brain (external anatomy)
a. parietal lobe
b. occipital lobe
c. cerebellum
d. frontal lobe
e. temporal lobe

FIG. **4-3** Brain (sagittal and coronal sections)
a. pituitary gland
b. pons
c. spinal cord
d. cerebellum
e. brain stem

FIG. **4-4** Brain (meninges and spinal fluid)
a. scalp
b. inner layer
c. dural sinus
d. arachnoid villus
e. outer layer
f. skull bone
g. dura mater

h. arachnoid
i. subarachnoid space
j. pia mater
k. cerebral cortex
l. falx cerebri

FIG. **4-5** Spinal cord (cross-sections)
a. central canal
b. ventral root
c. spinal nerve
d. white matter
e. gray matter
f. dorsal root
g. pia mater
h. dura mater

FIG. **4-6** Nerves of the spine
a. cranial nerves
b. cerebellum
c. cervical spinal nerves
d. brachial plexeus
e. thoracic spinal nerves
f. lumbar spinal nerves
g. sacral spinal nerves

FIG. **4-7** Cranial nerves
a. optic
b. trochlear
c. abducens
d. facial
e. vagus
f. accessory
g. olfactory
h. oculomator
i. trigeminal
j. facial
k. hypoglossal

UNIT 5 The Eye

FIG. **5-1** Structures of the eye (cross-section)
a. ciliary body
b. conjunctiva
c. cornea
d. iris
e. pupil
f. lens
g. ciliary muscle
h. vitreous body
i. retina
j. fovea centralis
k. retinal blood vessels
l. optic nerve
m. macula
n. choroid
o. sclera

Answer Key

UNIT 6 The Ear

FIG. **6-1** Structures of the ear
(inner bones)
a. anterior canal
b. posterior canal
c. lateral canal
d. cochlea
e. organ of Corti
f. semicircular canals
g. oval window
h. round window

FIG. **6-2** Structures of the ear (outer
structures)
a. pinna
b. temporal bone
c. semicircular canals
d. inner ear
e. cochlea
f. eustachian tube
g. vestibule
h. eardrum
i. auditory canal
j. outer ear (antihelix)

UNIT 7 The Nose, Mouth, and Throat

FIG. **7-1** The nose, mouth, and throat
a. soft palate
b. pharynx
c. epiglottis
d. esophagus
e. nasal cavity
f. hard palate
g. tongue
h. mandible
i. vocal cords
j. trachea

FIG. **7-2** Structures of the tongue
a. root
b. body
c. epiglottis
d. lingual tonsils
e. bitter
f. sour
g. papillae
h. salt
i. sweet

FIG. **7-3** Throat structure (cross-section)
a. hyoid bone
b. cricothyroid ligament
c. cricoid cartilage
d. epiglottis
e. thyrohyoid membrane
f. thyroid cartilage
g. trachea cartilage

UNIT 8 Teeth

FIG. **8-1** Types of teeth
a. molars
b. premolars
c. canines
d. incisors
e. canines
f. premolars
g. molars
h. molars
i. premolars
j. canines
k. incisors
l. canines
m. premolars
n. molars

FIG. **8-2** Tooth structure
a. crown
b. neck
c. root
d. enamel
e. dentin
f. pulp cavity
g. gingiva
h. alveolar bone
i. root canal

UNIT 9 The Heart

FIG. **9-1** Basic structure and circulation
of the heart
a. right atrium
b. right coronary artery
c. anterior cardiac veins
d. left coronary artery
e. left auricle
f. circumflex artery
g. great cardiac

FIG. **9-2** Cross-section of the heart
a. left pulmonary artery
b. right pulmonary artery
c. superior vena cava
d. right atrium
e. pulmonary semilunar valve
f. right AV valve
g. right ventricle
h. inferior vena cava
i. papillary muscles
j. aortic arch
k. aorta
l. left pulmonary veins
m. right pulmonary veins
n. left atrium
o. left AV valve
p. aortic semilunar valve
q. left ventricle

r. intraventricular septum
s. descending aorta

FIG. **9-3** How the heart beats (cardiac cycle)
Heartbeat sequence
a. Relaxation blood fills the atria
b. Atrial systole and ventricular diastole
c. Ventricular systole
d. Ventricles full tricuspid and mitral valves close

UNIT 10 The Circulatory System

FIG. **10-1** Types of blood vessels (arterioles)
a. endothelium
b. internal elastic lamina
c. tunica media
d. external elastic lamina
e. external elastic lamina
f. arteriole
g. collagen & elastic fibers

FIG. **10-2** Types of blood vessels (venous)
a. endothelium
b. valve cusp
c. tunica interna
d. tunica media
e. tunica externa
f. venule

FIG. **10-3** How the system works (arterioles)
a. external carotid
b. brachial cephalic
c. brachial
d. renal
e. abdominal aorta
f. radial
g. common iliac
h. popliteal
i. anterior tibial
j. internal carotid
k. common carotid
l. subclavian
m. axillary
n. celiac trunk
o. superior mesenteric
p. ulnar
q. femoral
r. posterior tibial

FIG. **10-4** How the system works (venous)
a. brachiocephalic
b. superior vena cava
c. brachial
d. inferior vena cava
e. renal
f. radial
g. common iliac
h. greater saphenous

i. posterior tibial
j. internal jugular
k. subclavian
l. axillary
m. cephalic
n. hepatic
o. ulnar
p. femoral
q. popliteal
r. anterior tibial

UNIT 11 The Lungs

FIG. **11-1** Basic lung structures
a. clavicle
b. apex right lung
c. mediastinum
d. intact lung
e. inferior lobe
f. diaphragm
g. larynx
h. trachea
i. primary bronchus
j. secondary bronchus
k. tertiary bronchus

UNIT 12 The Lymphatic System and Spleen

FIG. **12-1** Overview
a. palatine tonsil
b. thymus gland
c. axillary lymph node
d. spleen
e. iliac lymph node

UNIT 13 The Endocrine System

FIG. **13-1** Types of endocrine glands
a. hypothalamus
b. pineal gland
c. parathyroid gland
d. pituitary gland
e. thyroid gland
f. thymus gland
g. adrenal gland
h. pancreas
i. ovary
j. testis

UNIT 14 The Digestive System

FIG. **14-1** Basic digestive system structure
a. oral cavity
b. liver
c. pancreas
d. appendix
e. salivary gland

Answer Key

f. pharynx
g. esophagus
h. stomach
i. large intestine
j. small intestine
k. rectum
l. anus

FIG. **14-2**   Stomach (cross-section)

a. pyloric sphincter
b. duodenum
c. pylorus
d. esophagus
e. fundus
f. body

FIG. **14-3**   Small and large intestines (cross-section)

a. transverse colon
b. ileum
c. cecum
d. appendix
e. duodenum
f. descending colon
g. sigmoid colon
h. rectum
i. anus

UNIT 15   The Urinary System

FIG. **15-1**   Basic urinary system structure

a. right kidney
b. bladder
c. urethra
d. left kidney
e. ureter

FIG. **15-2**   Cross-section of kidney

a. cortex
b. renal artery
c. renal vein
d. renal pelvis
e. ureter
f. calyx
g. renal pyramid
h. renal column

UNIT 16   Male Reproductive System

FIG. **16-1**   Basic structure

a. seminal vesicle
b. ejaculatory duct
c. rectum
d. bulbourethral gland
e. epididymis
f. testes
g. urinary bladder
h. ductus deferens

i. symphysis pubis
j. prostate gland
k. urethra
l. penis
m. glans penis
n. prepuce
o. scrotum

UNIT 17   Female Reproductive System

FIG. **17-1**   Basic structure (cross-section or ventral view)

a. uterus
b. rectum
c. coccyx
d. sacrum
e. anus
f. labium minora
g. labium majora
h. ovary fimbriae
i. ovary
j. uterine tube
k. urinary bladder
l. symphysis pubis
m. urethra
n. clitoris
o. vagina

FIG. **17-2**   Posterior view

a. fallopian tube
b. ovarian ligament
c. vagina
d. ovary
e. uterus

FIG. **17-3**   External genitalia

a. labia majora
b. urethral orifice
c. vaginal orifice
d. anus
e. mons pubis
f. prepuce
g. clitoris
h. labia minora
i. vestibule

FIG. **17-4**   Breast (Cross-section)

a. mammary ducts
b. areola
c. nipple
d. mammary gland
e. adipose tissue
f. pectoralis major
g. ribs
h. intercostals muscles

Jasodha . Naidoo @ hunter. Co

(1) Bell ringer: week of Nov . 30

(2) Physiology lab exam: Dec 8 - 18
(with lecture final exam)